MCQs in Orthopaedics and T

To Angela

MCQs in Orthopaedics and Trauma

G.S.E. Dowd
MB ChB MD MChOrth FRCS(Eng)
Senior Lecturer in Orthopaedics,
The Institute of Orthopaedics,
University of London, UK
Honorary Consultant in Orthopaedics and Trauma,
Royal National Orthopaedic Hospital,
London, UK

Churchill Livingstone
EDINBURGH LONDON MELBOURNE AND NEW YORK 1987

CHURCHILL LIVINGSTONE
Medical Division of Longman Group UK Limited

Distributed in the United States of America by Churchill Livingstone Inc., 1560 Broadway, New York, N.Y. 10036, and by associated companies, branches and representatives throughout the world.

First published 1987

ISBN 0-443-03372-2

British Library Cataloguing in Publication Data
Dowd, G.S.E.
MCQs in orthopaedics and trauma.
1. Orthopedia — Problems, exercises, etc.
2. Wounds and injuries — Problems, exercises, etc.
I. Title
617'.3'0076 RD732.6

Library of Congress Cataloging in Publication Data
Dowd, G.S.E.
MCQs in orthopaedics and trauma.
1. Orthopedia — Examinations, questions, etc.
2. Wounds and injuries — Examinations, questions, etc.
I. Title. [DNLM: 1. Orthopedics — examination questions.
2. Wounds and Injuries — examinations questions.
WE 18 D745m]
RD732.6.D68 1986 617.3'0076 86-13519

Produced by Longman Singapore Publishers (Pte) Ltd.
Printed in Singapore.

Preface

The purpose of this multiple choice question book is two-fold. It provides examples of questions that may be set in final MB examinations and it is also designed to act as a useful method of revision. The book is divided into two sections, orthopaedics and trauma. Within the sections, the questions are broad-based and have been randomly allocated. While the majority of questions should be answered correctly by the average competent student, some questions have been set at a more difficult level. The answer sections to each question are aimed at providing basic facts on the subject presented, but are not designed to be comprehensive. In a section where further information is needed, the reader should refer to a standard textbook.

It is hoped that the book will provide the student with an introduction to the type of questions that may arise in multiple choice examinations and at the same time allow self-assessment in the specialty with the aim that this will improve his knowledge of orthopaedics and trauma. I have tried to remove any points of ambiguity, by requesting critical appraisal from registrars and other medical staff, but inevitably some may still arise. Eponyms have been used sparingly where their usage is common-place and providing their meaning is generally accepted.

I am most grateful to the publishers Churchill Livingstone for their help and co-operation in publishing this book and to Miss Barbara Smith for typing the manuscript.

London, 1987 G.S.E.D.

Contents

Orthopaedics

Questions (*Answers overleaf*)

1 Rheumatoid arthritis may be associated with

A early morning joint stiffness
B ulnar deviation of the metacarpophalangeal joints
C a negative latex test
D rupture of extensor tendons of the hands
E instability of the atlanto-axial joint on radiological examination

2 Spastic cerebral palsy has the following features

A Increased muscle tone associated with a lack of voluntary control
B In the lower limb, the hip is flexed, the knee extended and the ankle plantar flexed
C In the upper limb, the elbow is flexed, the forearm pronated, the wrist flexed and the thumb adducted
D The mental state is invariably impaired
E Defective vision and deafness may retard the child's progress

Answers

1 A **True**
B **True**
C **True**
D **True**
E **True**

Rheumatoid arthritis, a disease affecting the synovial lining of joints and accompanied by extra-articular manifestations including subcutaneous nodules and infiltration of tendons and synovial sheaths, is often heralded by a history of early morning joint stiffness especially in the hands. Involvement of the metacarpophalangeal joints with joint laxity, ulnar subluxation of the extensor tendons and the effects of gravity on the hand in many functional position, results in ulnar deviation. Laxity of the joints at the atlanto-axial level results in instability. Many patients with well established rheumatoid have a negative latex fixation test. Rupture of extensor tendons usually occurs at the wrist due to infiltration by hypertrophied synovial tissue and constriction by the extensor retinaculum.

2 A **True**
B **False**
C **True**
D **False**
E **True**

Cerebral palsy is a term encompassing several clinical disorders in which the main feature is a primary lesion within the brain. It is most frequently caused by a difficult labour resulting in cerebral anoxia or haemorrhage, but also by developmental anomalies prenatally and infections or trauma postnatally. When the damage involves the motor cortex the clinical features are those of an upper motor neurone lesion, including increased muscle tone with lack of voluntary control. The spasm and muscle imbalance may result in deformity which in the upper limbs is elbow flexion, forearm pronation, flexed wrist and adducted thumb. In the lower limb, the hip is flexed and adducted, the knee flexed and the ankle plantarflexed. Depending on involvement of other areas of the brain, there may be intellectual impairment, blindness and deafness.

Questions (*Answers overleaf*)

3 Osteosarcoma

A is most common in the second decade of life
B requires eradication of the bulk of the tumour before chemotherapy can be successful
C occurs most commonly around the knee joint
D can always be diagnosed on radiographs
E associated with pre-existing Paget's disease, carries a good prognosis

4 Osteochondritis dissecans is

A only a disorder of the knee
B usually found on the lateral side of the medial femoral condyle of the knee
C a local separation of bone and cartilage from a normal bed of bone
D a cause of a loose body in the knee joint
E always treated by excision of the loose fragment

5 Osteochondromata (multiple exostoses, diaphyseal aclasis)

A are benign, without the capacity for malignant change
B occur most commonly in the diaphyseal area of a long bone
C may be a cause of leg length inequality
D are usually larger clinically than radiologically
E develop with the distal end of the bony outgrowth directed towards the adjacent joint

Answers

3
- A **True**
- B **True**
- C **True**
- D **False**
- E **False**

Osteosarcoma, a malignant tumour arising from primitive bone-forrning cells occurs most commonly in the second decade of life, with a further peak in later life when associated with Paget's disease. Eighty per cent of cases occur in the upper tibia and lower femur. Diagnosis depends on radiological features together with accurate histological diagnosis by biopsy in all cases. For chemotherapy to be effective on microscopic secondary deposits, the bulk of the tumour must be removed by amputation of the limb or wide excision and prosthetic replacement. Prognosis in Paget's disease is poor despite recent advances in treatment.

4
- A **False**
- B **True**
- C **True**
- D **True**
- E **False**

Osteochondritis dissecans is a disorder of synovial joints in which an area of subchondral bone becomes avascular and separates, together with the adjacent articular cartilage, from its bed. If it completely separates it will become a loose body. Treatment at this stage depends on whether the fragment can be accurately replaced in its bed and fixed with a Smillie pin or whether it should be removed. The commonest site is the knee, but other joints including the elbow, ankle and hip may be affected.

5
- A **False**
- B **False**
- C **True**
- D **True**
- E **False**

Osteochondromata develop from the growth plate and with bone growth move into the metaphysis with the tip of the growth pointing away from the joint. They consist of a bony stalk and head, capped by cartilage. Since cartilage is radiolucent, the size of the swelling clinically will be larger than that present on radiological examination. Osteochondromata may present clinically as leg length inequality since they may interfere with skeletal growth. Very rarely, the cartilaginous part of the tumour may undergo sarcomatous change to a chondrosarcoma.

Questions (*Answers overleaf*)

6 Ollier's disease (multiple enchondromatosis) is
A a dyschondroplasia
B usually found to affect limbs bilaterally
C genetically inherited by an autosomal dominant gene
D associated with shortening and modelling abnormalities of long bones
E occasionally associated with the development of a chondrosarcoma

7 The following muscles are flexors of the wrist
A Brachioradialis
B Flexor carpi ulnaris
C Pronator teres
D Flexor digitorum profundus
E Flexor pollicis brevis

8 A Kellers operation for hallux valgus consists of
A excision of the metatarsal head
B simple excision of the bunion
C a displacement osteotomy through the neck of the metatarsal
D excision of the proximal third of the proximal phalanx, elongation of the extensor hallucis longus and removal of the medial bony prominence of the metatarsal head
E an oblique osteotomy through the shaft of the metatarsal

9 The carpal tunnel syndrome may be associated with
A diabetes
B supracondylar fracture
C rheumatoid arthritis
D syringomyelia
E acromegaly

Answers

6 A **True** B **False** C **False** D **True** E **True**

Olliers disease is a dyschondroplasia without a genetic inheritance in which masses of unossified cartilage remain within the metaphyses of long bones, usually unilaterally, and is associated with retarded bone growth and poor remodelling. Occasionally one of the tumours may undergo malignant change to a chondrosarcoma. Multiple enchondromata associated with soft tissue haemangiomata is called Maffuci's syndrome and when associated with intestinal polyps and soft tissue hamartomas is called Gardner's syndrome.

7 A **False** B **True** C **False** D **True** E **False**

The wrist flexors include flexor carpi radialis, the long thumb and finger flexors, flexor carpi ulnaris and the vestigial palmaris longus. Brachioradialis inserts into the radial styloid and has no effect on wrist movement. Pronator teres acts as a pronator of the forearm and flexor of the elbow. Flexor pollicis brevis arises from the flexor retinaculum and has no effect on wrist flexion.

8 A **False** B **False** C **False** D **True** E **False**

A Kellers operation, described by an American Army Surgeon in 1904 for hallux valgus, includes excision of the proximal third of the proximal phalanx, extensor hallucis longus elongation and removal of the bony medial prominence of the metatarsal head. Excision of the metatarsal head is called a Mayo's operation. Displacement osteotomies commonly used for hallux valgus include a Mitchell's osteotomy through the neck of the metatarsal and a Wilson's osteotomy which is an oblique osteotomy thorough the shaft of the metatarsal. The aim of both osteotomies is to produce realignment of the great toe and narrowing of the forefoot by displacing the distal fragment laterally.

9 A **True** B **False** C **True** D **False** E **True**

Carpal tunnel syndrome is caused by an irritation of the median nerve which is compressed within the tunnel created by the carpal bones and the flexor retinaculum. Most are idiopathic, but presumably may be associated with decrease in volume due to bony encroachment or synovitis. Predisposing factors include pregnancy and the pill, diabetes, rheumatoid arthritis and any other inflammatory disorder, acromegaly, myxoedema and following injury at the wrist including Colles fracture or the rare injury, lunate dislocation.

Questions (*Answers overleaf*)

10 Dupuytren's contracture has the following features

A Pain over the radial styloid made worse by extending the thumb against resistance
B Thickening and contraction of the palmar aponeurosis
C A history of liver disease in some patients
D It is commoner in women than men
E The development of fixed contractures of finger joints

11 Fibrous dysplasia of bone has the following features

A It may affect a solitary bone or there may be widespread skeletal involvement
B It may be associated with endocrine disturbances and cutaneous pigmentation
C The lower extremities are most frequently and extensively involved
D Malignant change is common
E It never affects the skull

12 Paget's disease of bone is associated with

A deafness and blindness
B normal blood plasma biochemistry
C pathological fractures
D pain relief when treated with calcitonin
E an abnormality of collagen synthesis

Answers

10 A **False**
B **True**
C **True**
D **False**
E **True**

Dupuytrens contracture is characterised by thickening and contracture within the palmar aponeurosis resulting, in the early stages, with nodules in the palm and subsequently with fixed flexion contracture mainly of the little and ring fingers. The disease is usually idiopathic but may be associated with epilepsy, liver disease and trauma. It is commoner in men than women. Pain and tenderness over the radial styloid is called De Quervain's synovitis in which the fibrous sheath over the extensor pollicis brevis and abductor pollicis longus is thickened resulting in a constriction of the tendons.

11 A **True**
B **True**
C **True**
D **False**
E **False**

Fibrous dysplasia is a skeletal disorder in which bone is replaced by fibrous tissue. It may occur in a monostotic or polyostotic form. The cause is unknown. The disorder affects all major long bones especially in the lower limbs and commonly the skull. If associated with cutaneous pigmentation and endocrine disturbances, including sexual precocity in females, it is called Albright's syndrome. Marked deformity of bone may occur. Blood investigations are normal.

12 A **True**
B **False**
C **True**
D **True**
E **False**

Paget's disease of bone is characterised by thickening, softening and deformity, with recalcification and hardening of bone. The cause is unknown. It affects the skull and may result in bony encroachment of the foramina resulting in blindness and deafness. When it affects the long bones there may be bowing and subsequent pathological fractures. Vertebral involvement may result in spinal cord symptoms. Serum calcium and phosphate are normal, but the alkaline phosphatase is often very high. Urinary hydroxyproline excretion is raised due to the high bone matrix turnover. Calcitonin therapy does relieve pain in many patients, but often symptoms recur on stopping treatment. Diphosphonates have also been used to decrease bone turnover.

Questions (*Answers overleaf*)

13 Osteoid osteoma

- **A** consists of an area of dense cortical bone thickening with a central lucent area, the nidus
- **B** classically produces pain relieved by aspirin
- **C** occasionally becomes malignant
- **D** may show up on a technetium 99m bone scan when not obvious on routine radiographs
- **E** is treated by excision of the cortical thickening and the nidus

14 Concerning the menisci of the knee

- **A** A tear usually occurs through the length of the meniscus
- **B** Radiological signs of degenerative arthritis in the knee occur in upto 50% of patients 10 years following a total meniscectomy
- **C** One of the functions of the meniscus is to improve lubrication of the knee joint
- **D** Meniscal tears are usually associated with a twisting injury to the knee
- **E** Tears of the meniscus occur more frequently on the lateral side of the knee than the medial

Answers

13 A **True**
B **True**
C **False**
D **True**
E **True**

Osteoid osteoma, a benign lesion of bone with an unknown aetiology, classically presents with continuous aching pain, often worse at night and relieved by aspirin. There may be localised tenderness and thickening at the site of pain when the bone involved is subcutaneous. The radiographic features are bone sclerosis with thickening of the cortex together with a central lucency, the nidus. Visualisation of the nidus may require tomography. Occasionally, the lesion may not be apparent on radiographs, but a technetium 99m bone scan will demonstrate a 'hot spot'. A complete cure will result from excision of the sclerotic bone and nidus. Malignant change is not a recognised complication.

14 A **True**
B **True**
C **True**
D **True**
E **False**

The menisci have several functions in the knee. They act as a small part of the stabilising mechanism between femur and tibia. They facilitate lubrication of the joint and play an important role in load-bearing and distribution of load between femur and tibia. Most meniscal tears are associated with twisting injuries of the knee. They produce tears through the length of the meniscus either at the periphery or within the body along the line of fibre orientation. Since the lateral meniscus has a greater mobility than the medial, it is injured less frequently. Total meniscectomy is no longer believed to be an innocuous procedure since it is associated with a high percentage of degenerative change in the long term.

Questions (*Answers overleaf*)

15 A patient aged 65 years had a total hip replacement fixed with bone cement 3 years previously and now complains of aching pain in the groin associated with a limp when exercising. The following procedures may aid diagnosis

A Antero-posterior radiographs of the hip
B Blood cultures
C Aspiration of the hip joint
D A technetium 99m bone scan
E Rest in a spica for 6 weeks

16 Haemophilia

A has an autosomal recessive inheritance
B is caused by a deficiency of factor VIII, antihaemophilic factor
C most commonly affects the knee, elbow and and ankle joints
D results in a decreased prothrombin time, but normal clotting time
E may result in osteoarthritis of the hip joint which can be successfully treated by a total hip replacement

17 A 13 year old boy develops a painful, swollen knee joint without a history of trauma. He is febrile and has a tachycardia. Which of the following investigations would aid diagnosis of an acute septic arthritis?

A Chest radiograph
B Blood cultures
C Aspiration of the joint
D Erythrocyte sedimentation rate and white cell count
E A bone scan

Answers

15 A **True** B **False** C **True** D **True** E **False**

The two commonest causes for pain and a limp following a total hip replacement are mechanical loosening of the prosthesis or low grade infection. A radiographic assessment may show loosening of the prosthesis or a fracture through the stem or cement. Blood cultures are not likely to reveal an organism unless the patient has a pyrexia. Aspiration of the hip under radiographic control may produce fluid which can be cultured for both aerobes and anaerobes, and it may be combined with an arthrogram to demonstrate loosening. A technetium 99m bone scan may show increased uptake in both mechanical loosening or infection. A gallium scan may differentiate between the two since it is taken up by leucocytes. Rest in a spica is unlikely to be a diagnostic aid since it will not stop mechanical loosening and will not eradicate subacute infection.

16 A **False** B **True** C **True** D **False** E **True**

Haemophilia is a disorder of blood coagulation due to a deficiency in Factor VIII. It is transmitted as a sex-linked recessive, although about one-third of all cases are sporadic. The clotting time is increased but the prothrombin time and bleeding time are normal. The most commonly affected joints are hinge joints such as the knee, elbow and ankle with the wrist, hip, shoulder, hand and foot being infrequently involved. Elective surgery, such as joint replacement and arthrodesis for chronic haemophilic arthropathy, is now possible providing medical and laboratory expertise is available to monitor factor VIII levels during replacement therapy.

17 A **False** B **True** C **True** D **True** E **True**

Radiographs of the knee are unlikely to show any abnormality in the acute stage. However, they are useful as a base-line for reference and should be taken as a routine. Blood cultures may identify the infecting organism in some cases and aspiration of the joint may produce turbid fluid which can be sent for microscopy and bacteriological culture. The erythrocyte sedimentation rate and white cell count will be raised in acute septic arthritis and are useful in monitoring the effect of treatment. A bone scan may be useful, since it may demonstrate a focal lesion in the adjacent femur or tibia, but it is not essential for diagnosis.

Questions (*Answers overleaf*)

18 Neurofibromatosis (Von Recklinghausen's disease) may present with

A leg length inequality
B pseudarthrosis of the tibia
C a rigid scoliosis
D dislocated hips
E mental deficiency

19 Neuropathic joints may be associated with the following conditions

A Achondroplasia
B Syringomyelia
C Syphilis
D Septic arthritis
E Diabetes

20 Multiple myeloma

A arises from the plasma cells within the bone marrow
B may present with a macrocytic anaemia associated with bone pain
C can be confirmed by histological examination of a marrow biopsy
D may cause hypercalcaemia
E produces the classical radiological feature of small punched-out areas especially in the long bones, ribs and skull

Answers

18 A **True** B **True** C **True** D **False** E **False**

Neurofibromatosis is a disease in which there are multiple tumours within the peripheral nerves. The neurofibromas are composed of masses of fibrous and fatty tissue. It has an autosomal dominant inheritance. It may present with leg length inequality due to gigantism of one limb. It is associated with pseudarthrosis of the tibia in children, soft tissue tumours, café-au-lait skin pigmentation and scoliosis. Occasionally the swellings within the peripheral nerves may undergo sarcomatous change.

19 A **False** B **True** C **True** D **False** E **True**

Neuropathic joints (Charcot joints) are those in which pain and position sense is absent or markedly diminished. As a result, the joints become deranged and develop degenerative changes. Underlying conditions include syphilis, diabetes, leprosy, congenital indifference to pain and in the upper limbs, syringomyelia. Multiple injections of hydrocortisone into a joint are also said to produce features of a Charcot joint.

20 A **True** B **False** C **True** D **True** E **True**

Multiple myeloma is a malignant tumour of bone marrow, arising from plasma cells. It involves the long bones, ribs, vertebral bodies, pelvic bones and skull, producing a radiological picture of multiple small radiolucent 'punched-out' areas. The patient may have a microcytic anaemia, feel unwell, have bone pain or develop chest infections. Diagnosis depends on radiological changes, immunophoresis showing abnormal globulins and marrow biopsy. The erythrocyte sedimentation rate may be very high and serum calcium may be raised due to increased bone destruction. Urine testing may demonstrate Bence-Jones protein.

Questions (*Answers overleaf*)

21 Ankylosing spondylitis

A is a chronic inflammation, progressing slowly to bony ankylosis of the joints of the spinal column and occasionally major limb joints
B occurs more commonly in young men than women
C often affects the small joints of the hands and feet
D is associated with a raised erythrocyte sedimentation rate, but otherwise a normal blood biochemistry
E affects the costo-vertebral joints resulting in decreased chest expansion

22 Acute osteomyelitis in children

A usually affects the diaphysis of long bones
B can be confirmed in the early stages by radiological examination
C presents with pain, fever, local swelling and malaise
D can be cured by oral antibiotics for 7 days as an outpatient
E is most often a staphylococcal infection

Answers

21 A **True** B **True** C **False** D **True** E **True**

Ankylosing spondylitis is a chronic inflammatory condition progressing slowly to bony ankylosis of the joints of the spinal column. There is often fusion of the sacroiliac joints and the hip joints may also be affected. Chest expansion is often markedly limited due to involvement of the costo-vertebral joints. Men are more commonly affected than women, usually in the third decade of life. Haematological investigations are normal apart from a raised erythrocyte sedimentation rate. There is a strong association between HLA B27 and ankylosing spondylitis. Radiographic changes include fusion of the sacroiliac joints, squaring of the vertebrae and eventual calcification of the anterior spinal ligament (bamboo spine).

22 A **False** B **False** C **True** D **False** E **True**

Acute osteomyelitis in children usually develops in the metaphysis of the long bones and presents with pain, local swelling and later the classical signs of inflammation including redness and increased local temperature. The child will feel ill and have a pyrexia. Radiological investigations usually reveal no abnormality in the early stages but later periosteal elevation and osteoporosis may become apparent. The white cell count and erythrocyte sedimentation rate are usually raised. Blood cultures will reveal the organism in about 50% of cases, the commonest organism being *Staphyloccocus aureus.* Treatment is either immediate exploration of the bone and decompression or initial conservative therapy with intravenous antibiotics for 3 weeks with operative treatment withheld unless the infection fails to respond to therapy.

Questions (*Answers overleaf*)

23 In nutritional osteomalacia
- **A** the serum calcium is low or normal
- **B** the urinary calcium is normal or raised
- **C** the serum phosphate is low
- **D** the serum alkaline phosphatase is normal
- **E** bone biopsy will show inadequate mineralisation

24 Osteoporosis
- **A** is a disorder in which the composition of bone is normal, but there is an insufficient total amount
- **B** occurs following long-term steroid therapy
- **C** is demonstrated radiologically by decreased bone density and thinning of the cortices
- **D** is commonly seen after the menopause
- **E** may be associated with pain in the thoracic spine following vertebral collapse

25 In a soldier standing to attention with his knees fully extended
- **A** the rectus femoris and ligamentum patellae will be tight
- **B** the popliteus muscle will be contracted to maintain the knee in a locked position
- **C** the posterior capsule of the knee joint will be tight
- **D** the anterior cruciate will be lax
- **E** the femoral nerve must be intact to maintain the knee in the fully extended position

Answers

23 A **True** B **False** C **True** D **False** E **True**

Osteomalacia is a metabolic disease of bone in which there is deficient mineralisation of the bone matrix due to a lowered concentration of calcium and phosphorus in the body fluids as a result of impaired absorption from the intestine. The cause is lack of vitamin D in the diet. The serum calcium is usually normal or on the low side of normal since a decrease in the serum calcium stimulates the parathyroids to produce parathormone which in turn mobilises calcium from bone. The phosphate is low and the alkaline phosphatase is raised due to increased bone turnover. Bone biopsy will show thinned trabeculae with marked osteoclastic activity and osteoid seams.

24 A **True** B **True** C **True** D **True** E **True**

Osteoporosis is a bone disorder in which the quality of the bone is normal, but the total volume decreased. It may be associated with prolonged bedrest and fracture immobilisation, endocrine disorders including thyrotoxicosis, Cushings syndrome and following the menopause. Other causes which may alter the state of bone include malabsorption syndromes and malnutrition. Haematological investigations are normal in idiopathic cases or reflect the underlying cause. Radiographic appearances include the loss of definition in the trabeculae with an accentuation of the thinned cortical walls. There may be pathological fractures especially in the vertebrae. The patient may be asymptomatic or suffer the symptoms of pathological fracture including spine or rib pain.

25 A **False** B **False** C **True** D **False** E **False**

With full extension of the knee, the anterior cruciate, collateral ligaments and posterior capsule become taught. Further extension of the medial femoral condyle is made possible by forward rotation of the lateral condyle around the tight anterior cruciate until the knee becomes 'locked'. In the 'locked' position, the knee is slightly hyperextended and is stable without the extensor pull of the vasti and rectus femoris. The popliteus muscle acts to 'unlock' the knee by pulling the posterior part of the lateral meniscus backwards and producing posterior rotation of the lateral femoral condyle by its insertion into an area near the lateral epicondyle.

Questions (*Answers overleaf*)

26 Which of the following statements concerning spondylolisthesis of the lumbar spine are correct?

A Spondylolisthesis caused by a defect in the pars interarticularis invariably causes symptoms
B The defect in the pars interarticularis is most easily viewed on an oblique X-ray of the spine
C It may be caused by degenerative changes in the posterior facet joints
D It may interfere with childbirth
E Neurological signs, caused by the slip of one vertebra on the other may require decompression of the nerve root and fusion of the affected vertebral segments

27 A diagnosis of acute gout is supported by

A sudden attacks of severe pain in the metatarsophalangeal joint of the great toe associated with redness and swelling
B a family history of the disorder
C aspiration of a swollen joint with the fluid demonstrating pyrophosphate crystals on polarised microscopy
D a rapid response to treatment by indocid
E a raised serum uric acid

28 In congenital dislocation of the hip

A boys are more commonly affected than girls
B the abnormality may not be diagnosed until the child begins to walk
C all hips in newborn babies should be examined routinely to exclude the abnormality
D ossification of the secondary centre in the upper end of femur will be delayed
E the affected limb will be shorter

Answers

26 A **False** B **True** C **True** D **True** E **True**

Spondylolisthesis is the term describing the displacement of one vertebral body upon another. Usually the upper vertebra slips forwards on the lower. The commonest cause under the age of 50 years is a defect in the pars interarticularis, the cause of which is debated between a congenital anomaly and stress fracture. It may be an incidental finding on radiographs and be asymptomatic. The oblique film demonstrates the outline of the 'Scots terrier', with the break seen in the neck formed by the pars interarticularis. Other causes of lumbar spondylolisthesis are degenerative with loss of facet joint stability, severe trauma, hypoplasia of the upper sacrum or neural arch of the fifth lumbar vertebra and pathological due to an underlying bony abnormality such as Paget's disease or osteogenesis imperfecta. A forward slip of L5 on the sacrum may decrease the diameter of the pelvic outlet and result in problems with childbirth. In severe cases, nerve roots may be entrapped and require decompression followed by fusion to stabilise the spine.

27 A **True** B **True** C **False** D **True** E **True**

Acute gout presents as severe pain and swelling with skin erythema, classically in the metatarso-phalangeal joint of the great toe but may also affect other joints including the knee, ankle or fingers. A family history is present in a third of cases. Aspiration of the joint may demonstrate uric acid crystals on polarised microscopy and serum uric acid estimation will be raised above normal. The acute attack will respond rapidly to indocid. The main differential diagnosis is acute septic arthritis.

28 A **False** B **True** C **True** D **True** E **True**

Congenital dislocation of the hip occurs more commonly in girls than boys and more frequently on the left than right side. The disorder can usually be identified soon after birth and therefore examination of the hips of all new-born babies is necessary. If the disorder is not diagnosed at birth, it is usually identified when the baby begins to walk and is noticed to have a limp. Radiographic changes at birth may not be obvious, since the secondary centre of ossification does not appear until about 6 months of age. In a dislocated hip, the ossification centre is usually smaller than the opposite normal side, Shenton's line will be broken and the acetabular roof will slope steeply.

Questions (*Answers overleaf*)

29 Pes cavus deformity of the foot may be associated with the following conditions

A Ankylosing spondylitis
B Spina bifida
C Rheumatoid arthritis
D Peroneal muscular atrophy
E Acromegaly

30 A 39 year old male with a suspected prolapsed intervertebral disc suddenly develops urinary retention. The following measures should be taken

A Bilateral leg traction with increasing application of weights
B Urgent radiculogram
C Conservative management including hourly monitoring of neurological signs until urinary function returns
D Preparation for urgent spinal exploration
E Insertion of an indwelling urinary catheter

31 A 5 year old child with a myelomeningocele has no function below the L3 nerve roots. The following are likely to be present

A Bladder paralysis
B Dislocated hips
C Flexion deformities of the knees
D Increased tone in the muscles of the lower limbs
E An intact sensory supply to the lower limbs

Answers

29 A **False** B **True** C **False** D **True** E **False**

Pes cavus is a deformity in which the longitudinal arch of the foot is excessively high. It is often associated with clawing of the toes. The cause in the majority of patients is obscure, but may be familial. It may be secondary to a neurological disorder including poliomyelitis, developmental abnormalities of the spine including spina bifida and diastematomyelia where a bar of bone or fibrous band splits the spinal cord. Hereditary disorders including Friedrich's ataxia and peroneal muscular atrophy are associated with pes cavus. Occasionally the deformity may be post-traumatic or related to congenital talipes equinovarus.

30 A **False** B **True** C **False** D **True** E **True**

Sudden urinary retention due to disc prolapse is a surgical emergency, since delay in treatment will result in permanent disability. The aim of management is to identify the level of the disc prolapse by radiculogram and to decompress the cauda equina by removal of the obstruction surgically. Insertion of a urinary catheter will be necessary to relieve bladder distension but should not detract from urgent treatment of the underlying problem. Careful neurological examination will reveal 'saddle' anaesthesia around the perineum since the sacral nerves supplying the bladder also innervate skin from their sensory branches.

31 A **True** B **True** C **False** D **False** E **False**

In a child with intact nerve roots to the third lumbar level, there would be some activity in the hip flexors and hip adductors innervated by L2 and L3 nerve roots. The effect of active flexion and adduction with paralysis of the extensors and abductors is to sublux and dislocate the hips. With active extensor activity without flexor activity in the knee, a recurvatum rather than fixed flexion of the joints would be expected. Bladder paralysis would be present since sacral nerve roots would not function. Sensation in the lower limbs would be grossly impaired since innervation is by nerve roots distal to the level involved. The neurological defect in spina bifida is lower motor neurone and the muscle tone would be flaccid in muscle innervated by nerve roots distal to L3.

Questions (*Answers overleaf*)

32 A man of 30 years presents with pain and stiffness in his back and limited chest expansion. The following investigations may be useful in supporting the diagnosis of ankylosing spondylitis

A Full blood count
B Erythrocyte sedimentation rate
C Radiographs of the sacro-iliac joints
D Radiograph of the chest
E Radiculogram

33 A 60 year old woman presents with malaise, weight loss, anaemia and limb girdle pain. X-rays show vertebral collapse and 'punched out' areas in the long bones and skull. The following are likely diagnoses

A Secondary deposits from breat carcinoma
B Osteoporosis
C Myeloma
D Rheumatoid arthritis
E Diabetes mellitus

34 Perthes disease of the hip is

A more common in girls than boys
B seen most commonly in the 10–15 year age group
C often associated with a history of injury
D a common cause of osteoarthritis in later life
E believed to be due to an inherited abnormality of bone metabolism

35 In congenital talipes equinovarus

A the ankle is plantarflexed and the forefoot adducted and everted
B the ankle is plantarflexed and the forefoot adducted and inverted
C there is an association with maternal oligohydramnios
D the calf may be underdeveloped
E operative treatment is invariably necessary at an early stage

Answers

32 A **False** B **True** C **True** D **False** E **False**

The symptoms of pain and stiffness in the spine associated with decreased chest expansion suggest a diagnosis of ankylosing spondylitis in a young man. The diagnosis would be supported by a raised erythrocyte sedimentation rate together with radiological changes, if present. These include 'squaring' of the vertebral bodies, obliteration of the sacro-iliac joints and in the late stage a 'bamboo' spine resulting from calcification of the anterior spinous ligaments.

33 A **True** B **False** C **True** D **False** E **False**

The presenting symptoms are suggestive of a neoplastic disease, confirmed by the radiological changes. Both secondary deposits and myeloma require further investigation. Osteoporosis is unlikely since systemic manifestations and radiological changes are not typical. The symptoms described may be associated with rheumatoid arthritis, but the radiological changes are not compatible.

34 A **False** B **False** C **False** D **False** E **False**

Perthes disease is a condition arising in childhood which is an abnormality of the upper femoral epiphysis probably due to repeated episodes of ischaemia. The precipitating cause of the ischaemia is unknown. It is seen four times more commonly in boys than girls and occurs most frequently between the age of 5 and 10 years. It is bilateral in about 15% of cases. The disease is an uncommon cause of osteoarthritis in later life.

35 A **False** B **True** C **True** D **True** E **False**

Congenitial talipes equinovarus may be classified into the postural type which rapidly corrects by manipulation and strapping and which may be related to prolonged malposition in utero, and the rigid type caused by a defect of fetal development. The deformities associated with congenital talipes equinovarus are inversion of the foot, plantarflexion of the ankle and adduction of the forefoot relative to the hindfoot. In 'postural' deformities, there is an association with maternal oligohydramnios and in utero moulding problems. In the 'rigid' type of deformity, there is underdevelopment of the calf muscles, but in the 'postural' type, the calf is normal. Most cases can be managed conservatively, but failure of correction within 6 to 12 weeks of life is considered by many to be an indication for operation.

Questions (*Answers overleaf*)

36 A 4 year old child develops pain in the hip joint with restriction of all movements, a pyrexia, high erythrocyte sedimentation rate and white cell count

A Traction should be applied to the limb until the pain has settled
B The child should be treated with oral antibiotics for 3 weeks
C Blood cultures should be taken
D The hip joint should be explored surgically
E A history of trauma should be sought

37 Trophic ulcers

A only occur in the sole of the foot
B may predispose to osteomyelitis of underlying bone
C are lesions of the skin associated with limb ischaemia
D most frequently occur under the heel of the foot
E are very painful

38 A chronic slipped upper femoral epiphysis

A is associated with decreased internal rotation, flexion, abduction and true shortening
B is seen more commonly in boys than girls
C occurs most commonly between 10–15 years of age
D should be treated by reduction under general anaesthetic
E rarely affects both hips

Answers

36 A **False** B **False** C **True** D **True** E **False**

The signs and symptoms are those of a septic arthritis. Irritable hip, a differential diagnosis, does not produce a pyrexia and high erythrocyte sedimentation rate. Septic arthritis of the hip should be considered a surgical emergency since delay in treatment will result in irreversible damage to the articular cartilage and femoral head. It may lead to growth arrest of the hip. The aim of treatment is to identify the organism, administer the appropriate antibiotic parenterally and also to decompress the hip by evacuating the pus. If there is doubt about the diagnosis, the hip should be explored. A conservative approach to treatment is not advocated by most authorities.

37 A **False** B **True** C **False** D **False** E **False**

Trophic ulcers occur as a direct or indirect result of abnormalities within the nervous system. While their pathogenesis is not completely understood, the main factor appears to be analgesia which allows repeated minor injury and excess pressure to pass unnoticed. While the majority of trophic ulcers occur in the sole of the foot overlying the metatarsal heads, they can occur in the fingers in patients with syringomyelia. The painless ulcers frequently become infected and subsequently the underlying bone may develop osteomyelitis. In the lower limbs, the causes include diabetes, tabes dorsalis, spina bifida with neurological deficit and peripheral nerve injuries.

38 A **True** B **True** C **True** D **False** E **False**

Chronic slipped upper femoral epiphysis occurs more frequently in boys than girls (3:1), in the 10–15 year age group. It occurs bilaterally in about a third of cases, raising the question whether prophylactic pinning of the unaffected hip should be performed. Most authorities advise against manual reduction of a chronic slip since it is usually ineffective and excessive pressure on the epiphysis may result in avascular necrosis. Usual treatment is by pinning the epiphysis in situ to prevent further slip and to perform an osteotomy at a later date to re-align the femoral head with the shaft. Clinically, the patient presents with aching pain in the hip or knee (referred pain) together with limitation of internal rotation, abduction and flexion.

Questions (*Answers overleaf*)

39 Cystic swellings in the popliteal fossa
- **A** do not occur in children
- **B** may be associated with osteoarthritis of the knee
- **C** occur in patients with rheumatoid arthritis affecting the knee joint
- **D** must be differentiated from popliteal aneurysms in adults
- **E** should always be excised

40 Loose bodies in the knee joint may be due to
- **A** osteochondral fractures
- **B** Osgood-Schlatter's disease
- **C** osteochondritis dissecans
- **D** osteoarthritis
- **E** synovial chondromatosis

Answers

39 A **False** B **True** C **True** D **True** E **False**

Cystic swellings within the popliteal fossa are not uncommon. Enlargement of the semimembranosus bursa occurs in children. In the adult, a 'blow out' from an osteoarthritic knee joint into the popliteal fossa may occur, producing a Baker's cyst. A similar cystic swelling may be associated with rheumatoid disease within the knee joint. Popliteal aneurysms occasionally occur in the older age group and may be diagnosed as a pulsatile swelling and confirmed by arteriogram. Treatment of cystic swellings obviously depends on the cause. In children, semimembranosus bursae may subside spontaneously but may be excised if they persist and cause discomfort. Baker's cysts may resolve if the pathology within the knee can be controlled. Anterior synovectomy usually results in spontaneous resolution of the popliteal swelling in rheumatoid arthritis, but if it remains may require excision.

40 A **True** B **False** C **True** D **True** E **True**

Loose bodies within the knee joint may consist of fibrous tissue, cartilage or bone and cartilage. Rarely they may be due to foreign bodies which have penetrated the knee joint. Fibrous loose bodies may result from osteoarthritis, tuberculosis and septic arthritis. Cartilaginous loose bodies may result from trauma including torn menisci. Osteo-cartilaginous loose bodies may also be caused by trauma including shearing fractures from the lateral femoral condyle caused by dislocation of the patella. Other causes of osteo-cartilaginous loose bodies are osteochondritis dissecans, detached osteophytes in osteoarthritis and synovial chondromatosis. Radiologically, fibrous and cartilaginous bodies are radiolucent unless they contain calcium. Osteo-cartilaginous bodies can be identified by their trabecular pattern. Osgood-Schlatter's disease is an extra-articular disease of the tibial apophysis.

Questions (*Answers overleaf*)

41 Avascular necrosis of the head of the femur is associated with
A gout
B Gaucher's disease
C fracture of the neck of femur
D steroid therapy
E diabetes

42 Which of the following are radiological features of idiopathic osteoarthritis?
A Osteoporosis of the bone adjacent to the joint
B Subchondral sclerosis
C Loss of joint space
D Osteophytes on the joint margins
E Subchondral cysts

43 Osgood-Schlatter's disease has the following features
A There is pain and tenderness over the swollen tibial tubercle
B It usually presents in early adolescence
C The erythrocyte sedimentation rate is raised
D Radiographic features include fragmentation of the anterior part of the tibial epiphysis
E It usually requires operative treatment

Answers

41 A **False**
B **True**
C **True**
D **True**
E **False**

Partial or total interruption of the blood supply to the femoral head resulting in avascular necrosis is associated with traumatic conditions including fracture of the neck of femur and dislocation of the hip. It is also associated with high dose steroid therapy, including treatment during renal transplantation and severe head injuries. It is also associated with Caissons's disease, liver disease, Sickle cell anaemia and Gaucher's disease in which there is an abnormality of lipid metabolism.

42 A **False**
B **True**
C **True**
D **True**
E **True**

The radiographic features of idiopathic osteoarthritis are: (a) narrowing of the joint space due to loss of articular cartilage, (b) subchondral bone sclerosis, (c) cyst formation in the subchondral area, (d) osteophyte formation at the joint margins, (e) altered shape of the joint. Osteoporosis is not a feature of idiopathic osteoarthritis, but may be associated with secondary joint involvement in diseases such as rheumatoid arthritis. In secondary arthritis other radiographic features may be present including evidence of a previous fracture or avascular necrosis from whatever cause.

43 A **True**
B **True**
C **False**
D **True**
E **False**

Osgood-Schlatter's disease is characterised by a painful swollen, tender tibial tuberosity. The pain is aggravated by kneeling and sporting activity, but is relieved by rest. It occurs between 10 and 15 years of age before closure of the tongue-like projection of the upper tibial epiphysis. There may be an association with injury, but this is not always the case. Radiographic appearances classically show a fragmented anterior part of the upper tibial epiphysis. All blood investigations are normal. Treatment is conservative with rest, and occasionally support with a plaster cylinder.

Questions (*Answers overleaf*)

44 Osteochondritis of the tarsal navicular (Kohler's disease) has the following features

- **A** It usually occurs in adolescence
- **B** Symptoms include mild pain and a limp, with swelling in the region of the navicular bone
- **C** Radiological changes include narrowing of the bone and increased density
- **D** The disease usually results in arthritic changes in adjacent joints
- **E** It is probably due to interference with the blood supply to the bone

45 Coxa vara

- **A** describes an abnormality of the upper end of the femur in which the neck-shaft angle is increased
- **B** may be a complication of intertrochanteric fractures
- **C** may be congenital in origin
- **D** increases the power of the abductors of the hip
- **E** will result in leg length inequality when unilateral

46 The following biochemical abnormalities are associated with primary hyperparathyroidism

- **A** Increased serum calcium
- **B** Low serum calcium
- **C** Low serum alkaline phosphatase
- **D** Raised serum phosphate
- **E** Low serum phosphate

Answers

44 A **False** B **True** C **True** D **False** E **True**

Kohler's disease of the tarsal navicular usually occurs between the ages of 3 and 6 years. Boys are more commonly affected than girls. The cause of the disease is unknown, but has been described as an osteochondritis, resulting from an interference with blood supply to the bone. The symptoms consist of pain and swelling over the tarsal navicular. The pain is aggravated by walking causing a limp on the affected side. Radiographs show fragmentation of the bone with subsequent spontaneous resolution.

45 A **False** B **True** C **True** D **False** E **True**

Coxa vara describes a deformity in which the neck-shaft angle of the proximal femur is decreased. It is commonly associated with malunion of intertrochanteric fractures. It occurs as a congenital abnormality which may be associated with shortening of the femur. Coxa vara may be caused by other abnormalities including slipped upper femoral epiphysis, rickets, Perthe's disease and Paget's disease. Biomechanically it decreases the power of the abductors. It results in loss of leg length on the affected side.

46 A **True** B **False** C **False** D **False** E **True**

Primary hyperparathyroidism is caused most frequently by a parathyroid adenoma or by hyperplasia or rarely by a carcinoma. In primary hyperparathyroidism, excess parathormone is produced. Its effect is to increase the serum calcium by mobilising calcium from bone and also by increasing the amount of calcium absorbed from the intestine. At the same time, phosphate loss is increased from the kidneys resulting in a low serum phosphate. Increased bone turnover results in a rise in alkaline phosphatase.

Questions (*Answers overleaf*)

47 Primary hyperparathyroidism may present with which of the following?

A Pathological fractures
B Peptic ulceration
C Pain and tenderness in the bones and muscles
D Muscle weakness
E Tetany due to increased sensitivity of muscle to contract

48 In the carpal tunnel syndrome

A pain and paraesthesia occur in the median nerve distribution of the hand
B symptoms do not usually affect sleep
C the 1st dorsal interosseous muscle is often wasted
D the thenar eminence muscles may be wasted
E nerve conduction studies may be useful to confirm diagnosis

49 Trigger finger

A occurs in children and adults
B is an abnormality in which the finger becomes fixed in flexion and requires either excessive extensor tendon activity, or manual reduction to allow the fingers to extend
C may be associated with rheumatoid arthritis
D may be associated with a palpable nodule in the flexor tendon
E may be treated by division of the proximal part of the fibrous flexor sheath

Answers

47 A **True**
B **True**
C **True**
D **True**
E **False**

Primary hyperparathyroidism is said to produce the classical clinical triad of 'bones, stones and abdominal groans'. Nephrocalcinosis and renal stones are the most common presentation due to deposition of the excess calcium in the renal tract. Bone changes of osteitis fibrosa cystica caused by bone resorption are uncommon. Bone pain is a feature of the disease and if the resorption is severe, pathological fractures may occur. Gastrointestinal problems producing the groans may include peptic ulceration and pancreatitis. Muscular weakness and hypotonia may be presenting symptoms. Tetany due to increased irritability of muscle is associated with hypoparathyroidism.

48 A **True**
B **False**
C **False**
D **True**
E **True**

The carpal tunnel syndrome results from compression of the median nerve as it passes under the flexor retinaculum at the wrist. Paraesthesiae in the median nerve distribution of the hand, often with radiation to the forearm is characteristic. The symptoms are frequently worse at night. Muscle weakness of the thenar eminence is usually a late feature, although the patient may complain of difficulty in picking up small objects. Nerve conduction studies may show delayed conduction along the median nerve across the wrist confirming diagnosis. In the early stages these tests may be normal.

49 A **True**
B **True**
C **True**
D **True**
E **True**

Trigger finger is a condition in which the flexor tendon becomes constricted by the surrounding fibrous flexor sheath of the finger. Often there is localised thickening forming a nodule within the tendon. With flexion of the finger, the nodule is released from the sheath and there is resistance to extension as the nodule is caught against the entrance to the flexor sheath. Extra effort may overcome the resistance and the finger extends with a sudden 'click'. Occasionally manual reduction is necessary to overcome the obstruction. Treatment is usually by division of the proximal part of the fibrous flexor sheath to allow free tracking of the flexor tendon.

Questions (*Answers overleaf*)

50 Concerning movement in the fingers

A The action of the intrinsic muscles is to flex the interphalangeal joints
B The long finger extensor tendons extend the metacarpophalangeal joints
C The intrinsic muscles flex the metacarpophalangeal joints
D The intrinsic muscles aid extension of the metacarpophalangeal joints
E Contraction of the dorsal interossei muscles results in adduction of the extended fingers towards the middle finger

51 Primary osteoarthritis is common in the following joints

A Hip
B Shoulder
C Metacarpophalangeal joint of the great toe
D Cervical spine facet joints
E Metacarpophalangeal joints of the fingers

52 'Locking' of the knee may be due to

A a loose body
B a pre-patellar bursa
C a torn meniscus
D osteoarthritis
E septic arthritis

Answers

50 A **False** B **True** C **True** D **False** E **False**

The intrinsic muscles (interossei and lumbricals), act to flex the metacarpophalangeal joints and to extend the proximal and distal inter-phalangeal joints by their insertion into the dorsal hood of the fingers. The dorsal interrossei act to abduct the fingers away from the middle finger with the fingers extended and the palmar interossei act to adduct the fingers ('PAD' and 'DAB'). The long extensor tendons act mainly to extend the metacarpophalangeal joints and to a lesser extent the inter-phalangeal joints.

51 A **True** B **False** C **True** D **True** E **False**

Primary osteoarthritis commonly affects the hip and knee joints. It also affects the carpo-metacarpal joints of the thumb and the metacarpophalangeal joints of the great toe. The lower cervical spine facet joints are frequently involved. The shoulder and ankle joints are rarely involved in the disease. The distal interphalangeal joints of the fingers are frequently affected with the development of Heberdens nodes (osteophytes) in comparison to rheumatoid arthritis which characteristically affects the metacarpophalangeal and proximal interphalangeal joints of the fingers.

52 A **True** B **False** C **True** D **True** E **False**

'Locking' of the knee to the surgeon means that the patient is unable to fully extend the knee. Frequently the patient uses the term to describe features including stiffness and other sensations which should not be described as 'locking'. Probably the most frequent cause of 'locking' is a torn meniscus in which the bucket handle lies within the intercondylar notch and stops full extension of the knee. Loose bodies may catch between femur and tibia to produce locking, as, for example, in osteoarthritis or osteochondritis dissecans.

Questions (*Answers overleaf*)

53 Giant cells tumours (osteoclastomas)

A occur before the end of growth
B are sometimes benign without the potential to metastasise
C produce a radiographic appearance of an eccentrically placed destructive lesion in the metaphysis which may reach the joint margin
D occur most commonly at the lower end of femur, upper end of tibia, lower end of radius and upper end of humerus
E may present with pain and gradually increasing local swelling

54 Tennis elbow

A is a disorder in which there is pain and tenderness over the origin of the extensor muscles of the forearm at the lateral epicondyle
B usually occurs following injury
C results in an exacerbation of symptoms when the wrist is flexed against resistance
D is associated with classical radiological changes
E is usually treated by an injection of hydrocortisone into the tender area

Answers

53 A **False**
B **True**
C **True**
D **True**
E **True**

Giant cell tumours (osteoclastomas) usually occur in young adults in which the growth plates have fused. Approximately one-third of tumours are benign and do not recur, a third are locally recurrent and a third are malignant producing metastases through the blood stream. The commonest sites are the lower end of femur and upper end of tibia, lower end of radius and upper end of humerus. The symptoms are pain associated with a gradually increasing local swelling. Occasionally a pathological fracture may be the first manifestation. Radiographic examination usually presents with the typical features of an eccentrically placed destructive lesion in the metaphysis which may reach the joint margin. Histological examination shows a tumour of bone containing many multinucleate giant cells within abundant oval or spindle-shaped stromal cells. Occasionally features of malignancy may be present.

54 A **True**
B **False**
C **False**
D **False**
E **True**

Tennis elbow is a well defined extra-articular condition in which there is pain and tenderness at the origin of the extensor tendons over the lateral epicondyle of the humerus. Despite many hypotheses, the cause is unknown. Symptoms can be exacerbated by forced extension of the wrist producing contraction in the extensor muscles. There are no radiographic changes in untreated cases. Treatment includes ultrasonics to the tender area or a hydrocortisone injection. Resistant cases, where the diagnosis is not in doubt, may be treated by stripping the extensor origin from its attachment to the lateral epicondyle.

Questions (*Answers overleaf*)

55 Anterior knee pain in adolescents may be associated with
A bipartite patella
B dislocation of the patella
C chondromalacia patellae
D bucket-handle tear of the meniscus
E plicae

56 Chondromalacia patellae
A is commoner in males than females
B occurs in the 10–30 year age group
C is a softening of the articular cartilage usually on the medial side of the patella
D should be treated by patellectomy at an early stage
E may be associated with patellar subluxation

Answers

55 A **True**
B **True**
C **True**
D **False**
E **True**

Anterior knee pain in adolescents may be due to chondromalacia patellae which may develop without an obvious cause or be secondary to recurrent subluxation or dislocation of the patella. Occasionally the pain may be due to a bipartite patella, with the small fragment found at the supero-lateral quadrant of the patella. Thickened synovial folds, plicae, may cause pain over the front of the knee as they 'snap' over the femoral condyle on flexion and extension of the knee. Bucket handle tears are unlikely to cause patello-femoral pain, the pain usually being localized to the side of the knee affected. In the older age groups, osteoarthritis is the commonest cause of patello-femoral pain, either in isolation or as part of a generalised knee disorder.

56 A **False**
B **True**
C **True**
D **False**
E **True**

Chondromalacia patellae, is a softening of articular cartilage most commonly on the medial side of the patella causing pain, joint effusions and a feeling of giving way. It is commoner in females and occurs in the 10–30 year age group. It is most commonly idiopathic, but may be related to patellar instability. It is said not to develop into osteoarthritis of the patello-femoral joint. Treatment is conservative initially including isometric quadriceps exercises. Realignment of the patella may improve symptoms in some cases with patellar instability. Only in very few cases with severe symptoms should patellectomy be considered and only after maximal quadriceps build-up.

Questions (*Answers overleaf*)

57 Primary osteoarthritis
- **A** is a disorder of articular cartilage which secondarily affects capsule, ligaments and subchondral bone
- **B** results in periarticular osteoporosis
- **C** is associated with a peripheral neuropathy and other systemic manifestations
- **D** occurs more commonly in men
- **E** is associated with synovial effusions caused by irritation of the synovial lining by products of articular cartilage breakdown

58 Protrusio acetabuli is associated with
- **A** avascular necrosis of the femoral head
- **B** Paget's disease
- **C** rheumatoid arthritis
- **D** intertrochanteric fractures
- **E** osteomalacia

Answers

57 A **True**
B **False**
C **False**
D **False**
E **True**

Primary osteoarthritis is a disease of articular cartilage, with other joint changes secondary to those of the cartilage. Many possible factors, resulting in damage to articular cartilage, have been postulated including biochemical abnormalities, microfractures of supporting bone, minor abnormalities of joint shape, body size and shape. Breakdown of articular cartilage, once initiated, usually continues until most of the joint is involved. Outgrowths around the periphery of the joint enlarge to become osteophytes. The subchondral bone becomes thickened, partly as a response to increased load bearing and also to crushing of the trabeculae. Subchondral cysts develop. Synovial irritation produces an outflow of synovial fluid, which is straw-coloured to produce an effusion. The capsule of the joint becomes thickened and contracted. It occurs with equal prevalence in males and females.

58 A **False**
B **True**
C **True**
D **False**
E **True**

Protrusio acetabuli is a disorder in which the femoral head sinks into the medial wall of the acetabulum. The first radiological sign is loss of the 'tear drop' which is the medial wall of the acetabulum seen on a routine antero-posterior radiograph of the pelvis. Further protrusion results in a bulge of the medial wall into the pelvis. The abnormality may be idiopathic when it is frequently bilateral (Otto's pelvis). Secondary causes include bone softening diseases, such as rheumatoid arthritis, osteomalacia and rickets, Paget's disease, osteoporosis, osteogenesis imperfecta and pelvic secondaries from malignant disease. Acetabular fractures may also be a cause of protrusio acetabuli.

Questions (*Answers overleaf*)

59 Sickle-cell disease
A is caused by an abnormality of haemoglobin synthesis
B is associated with chronic anaemia
C may result in infarction of the vessels supplying the upper femoral epiphysis
D may be successfully treated by long-term steroid therapy
E is seen most frequently in patients of European descent

60 Which of the following may produce periosteal elevation on radiographic examination in children?
A Osteosarcoma of the distal end of the femur
B Acute osteomyelitis of the distal end of femur
C Scurvy
D Battered baby syndrome
E Nutritional rickets

Answers

59 A **True** B **True** C **True** D **False** E **False**

Sickle-cell disease is caused by an abnormality in haemoglobin synthesis. It results in chronic anaemia because of the reduction in the life span of red cells. It also results in infarction of tissues including bone in conditions of reduced oxygen tension. It occurs in West Africans and those of African descent including West Indians. Genes for sickle cell disease are inherited from both parents. If one inherited gene is abnormal, the individual carries the trait but does not suffer from the disease. Abnormal genes from both parents are associated with the disease and consequent pathological abnormalities including limb pains, abdominal pains and anaemia. All patients at risk of the disease should be checked preoperatively so that the anaesthetist can avoid anoxic episodes during the anaesthetic.

60 A **True** B **True** C **True** D **True** E **True**

Periosteal elevation occurs in many skeletal disorders in children. The commonest cause is a fracture and can be seen on radiographs about a week after the injury when the radiolucent periosteum has laid down calcified intercellular matrix of collagen and mucopolysaccharide to form woven bone. Other disorders producing periosteal elevation include acute osteomyelitis, scurvy, and malignant bone tumours including osteosarcoma and Ewing's sarcoma. When there is an associated fracture, rickets produces periosteal elevation. The battered baby syndrome is associated with multiple fractures and is typified by varying stages of bone healing reflecting recurrent attacks on the child.

Questions (*Answers overleaf*)

61 Scoliosis is associated with the following conditions
- **A** Ankylosing spondylitis
- **B** Osteoid osteoma of the vertebral body
- **C** Leg length inequality
- **D** Neurofibromatosis
- **E** Hemivertebrae

62 Dupuytren's contracture of the hand is due to shortening or contracture of the following structures
- **A** The long flexor tendons
- **B** The palmar lumbrical muscles
- **C** The palmar interossei
- **D** The skin of the palm of the hand
- **E** The palmar aponeurosis

63 Dupuytrens contracture is associated with the following aetiological factors
- **A** Liver disease
- **B** Rheumatoid arthritis
- **C** Heavy manual work
- **D** A familial tendency
- **E** Diabetes

Answers

61 A **False** B **True** C **True** D **True** E **True**

A scoliosis is a lateral curvature of the spine. It may be associated with a kyphosis to produce a kyphoscoliosis. It may be postural, due, for example, to a unilateral short limb, or structural, in which there is rotation of the vertebrae producing, in the thoracic spine, a rib prominence. Structural scoliosis may be idiopathic, affecting girls more than boys or it may be due to bony, neurological or myopathic abnormalities. Examples of bony abnormalities are hemivertebrae. Neurological causes include poliomyelitis, neurofibromatosis and Friedrich's ataxia. Myopathic disorders include the many hereditary myopathies, for example Duchenne muscular dystrophy. Another cause of scoliosis is associated with pain from a local disorder, including osteoid osteoma or sciatica, which resolves providing the underlying disorder is treated early.

62 A **False** B **False** C **False** D **False** E **True**

Dupuytren's contracture, seen most commonly on the ulnar side of the hand, is due to contracture of the palmar aponeurosis. The earliest clinical sign is nodular thickening in the skin along the line of the flexor tendons. The aponeurosis extends fan shaped from the flexor retinaculum and sends slips into the fingers as far as the middle phalanges. As a result of contracture, the affected fingers develop a fixed flexion deformity. If the long flexor tendons were contracted then flexion of the wrist would relax the tendons and reduce the contracture. Intrinsic muscle contracture would lead to hyperextension of the interphalangeal joints. Contracture of the skin in the palm of the hand would not affect the fingers.

63 A **True** B **False** C **False** D **True** E **False**

Dupuytren's contracture is said to be associated with liver disease (alcoholic cirrhosis), epilepsy (in those patients taking epanutin), and a familial tendency. Although injury was described by Dupuytren as a factor there is still debate about the possibility. Heavy manual workers are no more at risk of the disease than sedentary workers.

Questions (*Answers overleaf*)

64 In facioscapulohumeral dystrophy

- **A** girls are more commonly affected than boys
- **B** it is usually transmitted as an autosomal recessive characteristic
- **C** the pectoralis muscle is frequently involved early in the disease
- **D** the patient often has difficulty whistling
- **E** most patients are chair-bound by the age of 10–15 years

65 The signs and symptoms in Marfan's syndrome may include

- **A** short stature for the patient's age
- **B** bilateral pes cavus
- **C** visual disturbances
- **D** a thoracic scoliosis
- **E** generalised muscle weakness

66 A swan-neck deformity of the finger has the following features

- **A** Hyperextension of the metacarpophalangeal joint, flexion of the proximal interphalangeal joint and extension of the distal interphalangeal joint
- **B** Flexion of the metacarpophalangeal joint, hyperextension of the proximal interphalangeal joint and flexion of the distal interphalangeal joint
- **C** It is frequently associated with rheumatoid arthritis
- **D** It is untreatable in patients with rheumatoid disease
- **E** It may be seen in normal individuals

Answers

64 A **False**
B **False**
C **True**
D **True**
E **False**

Facioscapulohumeral dystrophy affects boys and girls equally. It often passes from one generation to another as a Mendelian dominant character. One of the first features is the inability to whistle or close the eyes completely. The muscles of the shoulders and arms become affected and finally the muscles of the spine, hips and thighs. While some patients become chair-bound in their early teens, most are able to continue walking although with difficulty. Life expectancy may be normal.

65 A **False**
B **False**
C **True**
D **True**
E **True**

Marfan's syndrome is a growth abnormality, probably due to a biochemical disorder of collagen. It affects several systems including the skeleton, the cardiovascular system and the eyes. The patient is usually very tall and has arachnodactyly (long thin digits). There may be a severe scoliosis and the patient complains of a generalised muscle weakness. He may have a high-arch palate, hypermobile joints resulting in dislocating patellae and pes planus. The cardiovascular system may be affected by congenital heart disease, aortic dilatation and aneurysms. Ocular problems result from a lax or dislocated lens. The syndrome is inherited as a Mendelian dominant characteristic.

66 A **False**
B **True**
C **True**
D **False**
E **True**

Swan-neck deformity is frequently seen in rheumatoid disease but may occur in normal lax-jointed individuals. The deformity is one in which there is flexion of the metacarpophalangeal joints, hyperextension of the proximal interphalangeal joints and flexion of the terminal interphalangeal joints. In rheumatoid disease, synovial proliferation results in laxity of the proximal interphalangeal joints. Subsequent intrinsic tightness results in an irreducible deformity. In the early stages, synovectomy of the proximal interphalangeal joints with an intrinsic release procedure may produce a satisfactory result. A fixed deformity may require a proximal interphalangeal joint fusion with the joint flexed to approximately 30 degrees.

Questions (*Answers overleaf*)

67 Following a nerve injury
- **A** neurapraxia has the best prognosis for recovery
- **B** neurotmesis has the worst prognosis for recovery
- **C** axonotmesis describes complete transection of a nerve
- **D** axon regeneration following nerve repair occurs at the rate of about one millimetre a day
- **E** axon regeneration following nerve repair occurs at the rate of one centimetre a day

68 Which of the following are characteristic of the 'frozen shoulder' syndrome?
- **A** Males are far more commonly affected than females
- **B** Frequently all shoulder movements are decreased
- **C** There is usually a prodromal febrile illness
- **D** It is usually a self-limiting disorder
- **E** Radiological examination is normal

69 Knock-knee deformity (genu valgum) in children may be due to
- **A** normal lower limb development
- **B** rickets
- **C** chronic renal failure
- **D** osteogenesis imperfecta
- **E** Paget's disease

Answers

67 A **True** Nerve injuries have been classified into:
B **True** Neurapraxia, resulting in a transient physiological
C **False** block to conduction.
D **True** Axonotmesis, in which the gross anatomy of the
E **False** nerve is maintained but there is damage resulting in peripheral axonal degeneration.

Neurotmesis, in which the nerve is actually transected by an external force.

The average regeneration rate of a nerve following axonotmesis or successful repair of a transected nerve is about one millimetre a day.

68 A **False** Frozen shoulder is a disorder of unknown aetiology
B **True** in which there is generalised shoulder pain
C **False** associated with restriction of all movements. On
D **True** examination there is generalised tenderness and
E **True** restriction of all movements. Radiographs may show osteoporosis but no other abnormality. Blood tests are negative. The disorder affects males in equal numbers to females and patients are usually over 40 years of age. The disease is usually self-limiting, pain lasting 3–6 months and restriction of movement up to 2 years. Treatment includes hydrocortisone injections and physiotherapy or manipulation of the shoulder under anaesthetic.

69 A **True** Knock-knee deformity is a common normal stage of
B **True** development in the growth of lower limbs at about
C **True** 3–5 years of age. The deformity is usually
D **True** symmetrical and improves with growth. Before
E **False** accepting the deformity as developmental it is essential to exclude pathological disorders including rickets, renal disease, osteogenesis imperfecta and rare disorders including hypophosphatasia. Paget's disease does not occur in children.

Questions (*Answers overleaf*)

70 In which of the following is synovectomy indicated in rheumatoid disease?

- **A** In the knee, where synovial proliferation persists despite adequate conservative treatment and where articular cartilage damage is minimal
- **B** In the wrist, where prolonged synovial swelling along the extensor tendons will predispose to tendon rupture
- **C** In the wrist, where synovial proliferation in the carpal tunnel may produce symptoms of median nerve compression
- **D** In the knee, to ease pain in a severely destroyed joint
- **E** In the metacarpophalangeal joints which are swollen and painful despite conservative treatment

71 The internal rotators of the arm include

- **A** deltoid
- **B** pectoralis major
- **C** latissimus dorsi
- **D** serratus anterior
- **E** pectoralis minor

Answers

70 A **True**
B **True**
C **True**
D **False**
E **True**

Synovectomy, the removal of the lining of a joint, is a common procedure in rheumatoid surgery. Indications for the operation vary with individual surgeons, but there is a consensus for certain situations. In the knee, synovectomy is indicated when a boggy synovial swelling remains, despite conservative treatment, for longer than 6 months in a joint in which articular damage is minimal, With joint destruction, synovectomy is of little proven value. At the wrist, synovial proliferation in the carpal tunnel along the sheaths of the flexor tendons may cause compression of the median nerve. Decompression of the flexor retinaculum and synovectomy is indicated before irreversible nerve damage occurs. On the extensor surface, synovial hypertrophy may result in rupture of tendons and synovectomy should be performed as a prophylactic measure. In the hand, synovectomy is advised at the metacarpophalangeal joints where conservative treatment has failed to reduce the swelling and stiffness from synovial proliferation. Synovectomy of the interphalangeal joints has a debatable value with the risk of permanent joint stiffness.

71 A **False**
B **True**
C **True**
D **False**
E **False**

The pectoralis major and latissimus dorsi muscle which inserts into the floor of the bicipital groove, are major internal rotators of the shoulder. Subscapularis and teres major while acting as stabilisers of the shoulder also act as internal rotators. Serratus anterior arises from the ribs and inserts into the medial edge of the scapula. Pectoralis minor arises from the ribs and inserts into the coracoid process. Deltoid is essentially a shoulder abductor, while the anterior fibres act as a shoulder flexor.

Questions (*Answers overleaf*)

72 A 3 year old child presents with a limp and restriction of internal rotation and abduction of the hip. Which of the following may help to confirm the diagnosis of irritable hip?
- **A** A raised erythrocyte sedimentation rate
- **B** Improvement in hip movements following 48 hours of skin traction to the affected leg
- **C** A normal hip radiograph
- **D** A previous history of similar symptoms and signs
- **E** A pyrexia

73 A 10 year old child presents with spontaneous pain in the lumbar region. On examination there is restriction of spinal movements but no neurological abnormality in the lower limbs. Which of the following investigations may aid diagnosis?
- **A** A raised erythrocyte sedimentation rate
- **B** A bone scan
- **C** Routine antero-posterior and lateral radiographs of the lumbar spine
- **D** A radiculogram
- **E** A trial of oral antibiotics

Answers

72 A **False**
B **True**
C **True**
D **True**
E **False**

An irritable hip (transient synovitis) occurs in children and its cause is unknown. The child presents with a limp and pain in the hip and thigh. Examination reveals a restricted range of movement in the hip, especially internal rotation and abduction. The child is apyrexial and resting pulse rate is normal. All investigations are normal including radiographs. Bed rest and skin traction should result in early resolution of pain and improvement of range of movements. Full recovery occurs in several days in most patients but may take up to 10 days. Great care must be taken to exclude septic arthritis which may mimic an irritable hip in the early stages. Investigation in the latter will demonstrate a pyrexia, raised erythrocyte sedimentation rate and white cell count. Symptoms will deteriorate despite rest in septic arthritis.

73 A **True**
B **True**
C **True**
D **True**
E **False**

Symptoms of low back pain should be taken seriously in children, and fully investigated, since the underlying cause may include infection, tumours, spondylolisthesis and disc prolapse. Routine blood investigations will aid investigation of infection and tumours, including leukaemia. Radiographs may aid in the diagnosis of tumours, infections and bony abnormalities including spondylolisthesis. A technetium 99 m bone scan will be very useful to exclude infection or tumour and also occasionally an osteoid osteoma. A positive bone scan may be present in the early stages of an infection despite normal radiographs. Radiculography may be useful in identifying prolapsed intervertebral discs, which are uncommon in children. If infection is suspected, then full investigation and base line measurements of erythrocyte sedimentation rate and white cell count are necessary. Antibiotics should not be given as a therapeutic test, but only after investigation results in a firm diagnosis.

Questions (*Answers overleaf*)

74 Concerning cysts of the menisci
- **A** The medial meniscus is more commonly affected
- **B** The cyst may be related to a tear of the meniscus
- **C** Most cysts are soft in consistency
- **D** There may be a familial tendency
- **E** Most cysts subside spontaneously

75 The following are characteristic of De Quervain's tenosynovitis
- **A** Pain over the radial styloid made worse by actively extending the thumb
- **B** Pain over the ulnar styloid made worse by ulnar deviation of the wrist
- **C** A tender firm swelling over the radial styloid
- **D** Radiological changes on routine wrist radiographs
- **E** Spontaneous rapid resolution following a course of aspirin

76 Which of the following may cause shoulder pain?
- **A** A torn rotator cuff
- **B** Acute cholecystitis
- **C** Cervical spondylosis
- **D** Diaphragmatic pleurisy
- **E** Collapse of the 10th thoracic vertebra

Answers

74 A **False** B **True** C **False** D **False** E **False**

The aetiology of cystic menisci is disputed, but many are associated with horizontal tears of the menisci. The proposed mechanism of cyst formation is that the tear acts as a flap valve in which synovial fluid is compressed within the meniscus which expands the surrounding tissue to form a cyst. They occur most commonly on the lateral side of the knee and are usually small and firm. They are prominent at 30° of knee flexion and disappear on full flexion and extension. Most cysts do not subside and require operative excision. If there is an associated tear of the meniscus, the meniscus may have to be removed.

75 A **True** B **False** C **True** D **False** E **False**

DeQuervain's synovitis (stenosing tenovaginitis of the radial styloid) is a condition in which there is pain over the radial styloid associated with a palpable firm nodule in the fibrous sheath of abductor pollicis longus and extensor pollicis brevis tendons. Active resisted extension of the thumb exacerbates the pain. Radiographs in early cases are normal. The natural history of the disease is that it usually resolves spontaneously over a period of weeks. Persistent symptoms may be treated by one hydrocortisone injection or by surgical division of the fibrous sheath.

76 A **True** B **True** C **True** D **True** E **False**

Shoulder pain may be caused by a local disorder or by pain referred from a distant site. A careful history and examination should identify the cause. A torn rotator cuff lesion will produce local physical signs including tenderness and restricted shoulder movements. Acute cholecystitis may cause shoulder pain by irritating the right hemidiaphragm producing referred pain in the fourth cervical nerve distribution. Cervical spondylosis may present with generalised pain referred to the shoulder from an ill-defined and ill-understood cause or may be due to referred pain along the C4 and C5 dermatomes when foraminal encroachment irritates these nerves. Collapse of the tenth thoracic vertebra may irritate the ninth or tenth thoracic nerve roots which do not innervate the shoulder.

Questions (*Answers overleaf*)

77 Plantar fasciitis may be associated with the following conditions

- **A** Morton's metatarsalgia
- **B** Reiter's syndrome
- **C** Coronary thrombosis
- **D** Gout
- **E** Rheumatoid arthritis

78 Concerning the sheep agglutination test for rheumatoid arthritis

- **A** Sheep cells are coated with immunoglobulin IgG and reacted with the serum of the patient in varying dilutions
- **B** A negative test excludes the diagnosis of rheumatoid arthritis
- **C** The lowest titre of rheumatoid factor (IgM) in the patient's serum at which sheep cell agglutination occurs is measured
- **D** Tests for rheumatoid factor may be positive in normal elderly patients
- **E** Up to 80% of patients with rheumatoid arthritis have a positive test during their illness

79 In regard to synovium and synovial fluid

- **A** synovial fluid is an ultrafiltrate of plasma
- **B** normal synovial fluid contains about 1 to 4 g of protein per 100 ml of fluid
- **C** the normal knee joint contains about 50 ml of synovial fluid
- **D** the synovium consists of synovial cells at least 15–20 cells deep
- **E** glucose molecules are not found in normal synovial fluid

Answers

77 A **False** B **True** C **False** D **True** E **True**

Plantar fasciitis is a disorder in which there is pain and tenderness of the heel at the origin of the plantar fascia. The patient feels that he has a stone in his shoe. There is tenderness on palpatation of the sole at the insertion of the fascia at the calcaneum. Radiographs may be normal or show a spur of bone at the insertion of the plantar fascia into the calcaneum. Plantar fasciitis may be associated with Reiter's syndrome,gonorrhoea, ankylosing spondylitis, rheumatoid arthritis and gout.

78 A **True** B **False** C **False** D **True** E **True**

Rheumatoid factor is an anti-immunoglobulin found in most patients with rheumatoid arthritis. It is detected by agglutination with sensitised sheep cells or latex particles. The sheep cells are coated with 1gG and mixed with the patient's serum in increasing dilutions. The highest dilution (titre) at which agglutination occurs is measured. A positive titre varies with laboratories, but is usually about 1 in 32 or higher. Up to 80% of patients with symptoms and signs of rheumatoid arthritis have a positive test during their illness but a negative test does not exclude the diagnosis. A positive test to rheumatoid factor in low dilutions may occur in normal elderly patients.

79 A **True** B **True** C **False** D **False** E **False**

The synovium lines the joint cavity. It consists of synovial cells, one to two cells thick. Synovial fluid is an ultrafiltrate of plasma which also contains hyaluronic acid secreted by the synovial cells. Normal synovial fluid contains protein, mostly albumin and larger molecular weight proteins including fibrinogen. Small molecular weight substances such as glucose, amino acids and urate pass freely into the joint and their concentrations are equal to plasma. Normal knee joints contain about 0.5 ml of synovial fluid.

Questions (*Answers overleaf*)

80 Concerning the cervical spine in patients with rheumatoid arthritis

A Subluxation at the mid-cervical region is the commonest radiological abnormality
B Atlanto-axial subluxation can be identified by lateral flexion and extension views of the cervical spine
C Atlanto-axial subluxation may present with progressive long tract signs
D Atlanto-axial subluxation associated with pain requires urgent cervical fusion before neurological signs develop
E Erosion of the odontoid peg is more commonly a cause of atlanto-axial subluxation than annular ligament rupture

81 Sjogren's syndrome

A is the association of rheumatoid arthritis with dry eyes and mouth
B is the association of osteoarthritis with dry eyes and mouth
C may occur in about 10–15% of patients with rheumatoid arthritis presenting to hospital
D is due to blockage of the lacrimal and salivary ducts by stones
E can be treated by high-dose steroids

82 Psoriatic arthropathy

A tends to affect the terminal interphalangeal joints of the fingers in contrast to rheumatoid arthritis
B is often asymmetrical
C may present with a similar distribution to rheumatoid arthritis but with a negative rheumatoid factor
D is associated with pitting of the nails
E does not result in severe deformity in the hand

Answers

80 A **False** The cervical spine is frequently involved in
B **True** rheumatoid disease. The disease may affect
C **True** ligaments, joints, bones and disc spaces. Atlanto-
D **False** axial subluxation may occur in up to 25% of
E **False** rheumatoid patients and can be identified on lateral flexion-extension views. It is frequently due to laxity of the transverse ligament of the atlas and uncommonly to erosion of the odontoid peg. Most cases are asymptomatic or produce pain which can be relieved by a cervical collar. Patients with long tract or other neurological signs may require fusion to stabilise the segment. Other, less common problems are subluxation at the mid-cervical region and vertical subluxation in which the atlas protrudes into the foramen magnum.

81 A **True** Sjogren's syndrome is a symptom complex in
B **False** which rheumatoid arthritis is associated with dry
C **True** eyes (kerato-conjunctivitis sicca) and dry mouth
D **False** (xerostomia). The lacrimal and salivary glands
E **False** become infiltrated with lymphocytes and the duct linings undergo hyperplasia. No treatment is of value apart from application of methylcellulose eye drops and training in oral hygiene.

82 A **True** Psoriatic arthritis is a seronegative joint disorder
B **True** which often affects the terminal interphalangeal
C **True** joints and is asymmetrical. It may present with a
D **True** similar joint pattern to rheumatoid arthritis and
E **False** differentiating the two may be difficult. Pitting of the nails is associated with psoriatic arthropathy. About 1% of the population have psoriasis and of those, only 1% have arthropathy. Most patients have a mild non-progressive disease pattern, but occasionally a severe mutilating form may result in marked deformity in the hands (arthritis mutilans).

Questions (*Answers overleaf*)

83 Secondary osteoarthritis may be due to
- **A** congenital dislocation of the hip
- **B** an undisplaced, united fracture of the tibia
- **C** septic arthritis
- **D** acromegaly
- **E** Paget's disease

84 In normal articular cartilage
- **A** the framework consists of type II collagen fibres in a matrix of proteoglycan ground substance
- **B** the matrix is produced by fibroblasts
- **C** damage to the collagen fibres is rapidly repaired by the chondrocytes
- **D** the chondrocytes produce the matrix
- **E** the water content is small

Answers

83 A **True**
B **False**
C **True**
D **True**
E **True**

Secondary osteoarthritis may include the following as the primary disorder

(a) Congenital	— congenital dislocation of the hip
(b) Traumatic	— slipped upper femoral epiphysis
	— fracture of the neck of femur
	— torn menisci
	— loose bodies
(c) Inflammatory	— septic arthritis
	— tuberculosis
	— rheumatoid arthritis
	— psoriatic arthritis
(d) Metabolic	— gout
	— pseudogout (calcium
	— pyrophosphate)
	haemochromatosis
(e) Endocrine	— acromegaly
	— diabetes
	— Cushing's syndrome
(f) Others	— Paget's disease
	— haemophilia

84 A **True**
B **False**
C **False**
D **True**
E **False**

Articular cartilage is made up of a framework of type II collagen fibres in a matrix of proteoglycans (large macromolecules). Both the collagen and matrix are synthesised by chondrocytes which lie in lacunae within the matrix. The proteoglycan molecules, which consist of a protein core with chondroitin sulphate and keratin sulphate glycosaminoglycan side chains, have a great affinity for water which results in the turgidity and elasticity of cartilage. The chondrocytes show a poor response to injury since matrix turnover proceeds at a very slow rate and that of collagen is almost negligible.

Questions (*Answers overleaf*)

85 Radio-isotope imaging of bone by technetium 99m may be useful in diagnosing which of the following?
A Congenital dislocation of the hip
B Osteoid osteoma
C Carpal tunnel syndrome
D Malignant secondary bone deposits
E An infected intervertebral disc

86 Deformities of the hand associated with rheumatoid arthritis include
A ulnar deviation of the proximal interphalangeal joints
B decreased bulk of the thenar eminence
C boutonniere deformity of the interphalangeal joints
D inability to extend the interphalangeal joint of the thumb
E palmar subluxation of the metacarpophalangeal joints

87 Recurrent dislocation of the patella
A is commoner in boys than girls
B usually results in medial displacement of the patella
C may be treated by a realignment procedure of the patella
D should be treated by patellectomy at an early stage
E does not result in patello-femoral arthritis

Answers

85 A **False** B **True** C **False** D **True** E **True**

Technetium 99 m, with a half life of 6 hours, is injected intravenously 2–4 hours before the bone scan is carried out using a gamma camera. The bladder is emptied before scanning of the pelvis. Increased local blood flow is an important factor in deposition of tracers including technetium 99m. The technique is useful in detecting bone metastases that may not be seen on routine radiographs. It is also useful in bone and joint infection where it will show as a 'hot spot' even when routine radiographs may be normal.

86 A **False** B **True** C **True** D **False** E **True**

Deformities of the hand in rheumatoid arthritis are caused by ligament and capsular laxity, abnormal tendon pull or rupture, peripheral nerve involvement or damage to the bony architecture of a joint. Ligament and capsular laxity together with abnormal tendon pull results in ulnar deviation of the metacarpophalangeal joints. It also results in palmar subluxation of the metacarpophalangeal joints associated with hyperextension of the proximal interphalangeal joints and flexion of the terminal joints resulting in swan-neck deformity. Rupture of the central slip of the extensor hood and palmar drift of the lateral two slips results in a boutonniere deformity. Rupture of the long extensor tendon of the thumb results in inability to extend the metacarpo-phalangeal joint. Carpal tunnel syndrome, caused by compression of the median nerve by hypertrophied rheumatoid tissue, may result in loss of thenar muscle bulk.

87 A **False** B **False** C **True** D **False** E **False**

Recurrent dislocation of the patella is commoner in girls than boys. Frequently there is no specific history of direct injury to the knee. On flexing the knee during activity, the patella dislocates laterally and often reduces spontaneously. It usually occurs in the adolescent age group or in early adult life. Once dislocation occurs the patella tends to dislocate with increasing ease. Recurrent dislocation requires treatment to prevent further episodes of dislocation and to reduce the risk of patello-femoral arthritis. Operative treatment is aimed at re-aligning the patella in the femoral groove and this may be achieved by moving part of the patella tendon medially and by reefing the medial capsule of the knee and relaxing the lateral capsule (Roux-Goldthwait procedure).

Questions (*Answers overleaf*)

88 Predisposing factors in recurrent dislocation of the patella include

A flattening of the intercondylar groove
B abnormal quadriceps muscle pull on the patella
C a high-riding patella
D generalised ligament laxity
E genu varum

89 Normal bone

A consists of multiple units of bone lamellae surrounding a central canal containing osteoblasts and neurovascular bundles
B contains osteocytes which are involved in bone resorption and bone formation
C contains about 40% collagen in the intercellular matrix organic phase
D has crystalline hydroxyapatite in the inorganic phase
E contains about 65% inorganic, 25% organic constituents and only 10% of water by weight

Answers

88 A **True** B **True** C **True** D **True** E **False**

Recurrent dislocation of the patella is probably caused by a complex of factors in most patients. They include flattening of the intercondylar groove which can be seen on tangential radiographs of the patello-femoral joint. Familial joint laxity may be an important factor in some patients. A high-riding patella is associated with recurrent dislocation and it is interesting that the patella normally has a higher position in girls compared to boys. Genu valgum is said to be associated with dislocation, though there is debate, unless the deformity is severe. An abnormal quadriceps pull has been implicated, due to malpositioning of the patellar tendon insertion.

89 A **True** B **True** C **False** D **True** E **True**

The basic structural unit of bone is an osteon or Haversian system. It consists of circular lamellae around a central canal. Within the lamellae lie lacunae containing osteocytes. Within the central canal lie osteoblasts and neurovascular bundles. The osteocytes are involved in both bone formation and resorption. Osteoblasts, derived from mesenchymal cells, form osteoid, unmineralised bone matrix. Biochemically, bone consists of organic, and inorganic components and water. The organic component, consists of bone cells and intercellular matrix and comprises 25% of the wet bone weight. Ninety percent of the intercellular matrix consists of collagen fibres, the rest being other proteins and mucopolysaccharide complexes. The inorganic component, comprises 65% of the wet bone weight. It consists of crystalline hydroxyapatite calcium phosphate and other minerals including potassium, magnesium and fluoride. Ten percent of bone is water, in bone crystals and both intra and extracellular fluids.

Questions (*Answers overleaf*)

90 Hallux valgus

A is a deformity in which there is abnormal adduction of the great toe at the interphalangeal joint towards the middle of the foot
B may be defined as the abnormality in which the great toe is adducted at the metatarso-phalangeal joint with an angle greater than 30° when the axis of the 1st metatarsal is compared with the proximal phalanx
C rarely occurs in rheumatoid arthritis
D often results in pain over the prominent metatarsal head (bunion) when wearing shoes
E frequently results in pain due to osteoarthritis of the metatarsophalangeal joint

91 Carpo-metacarpal osteoarthritis of the thumb may be treated by

A excision of the trapezium
B fusion of the wrist
C fusion of the trapezio-scaphoid joint
D hydrocortisone injections into the joint
E fusion of the trapezio-metacarpal joint

92 Morton's metatarsalgia (interdigital neuroma) includes the following signs and symptoms

A Metatarsal pain on walking
B Pain most commonly between the great and second toe on compressing the forefoot
C A neuroma in the affected digital nerve
D Diminished sensation in the distribution of the nerve affected
E Relief of symptoms following excision of the neuroma

Answers

90	A	**True**	Hallux valgus may be defined as an abnormal adduction of the great toe towards the midline of the foot at the metatarsophalangeal joint. Normally the average angle between the long axis of the 1st metatarsal and the proximal phalanx is 10°. An angle greater than this may be defined as hallux valgus. The disorder can be idiopathic, familial and in some cases, related to abnormal shoe wear. It is commonly found in rheumatoid arthritis. Pain occurs because of degenerative change in the metatarsophalangeal joint, a prominent bunion or occasionally from the abnormal position of the sesamoid bones.
	B	**False**	
	C	**False**	
	D	**True**	
	E	**True**	
91	A	**True**	Osteoarthritis at the trapezio-metacarpal joint of the thumb is not uncommon, especially in women. In most cases symptoms are minor and respond to rest, physiotherapy or an injection of hydrocortisone. Joints which cause debilitating symptoms may be treated by fusion of the joint, excision arthroplasty of the trapezium or by a silastic replacement of the trapezium. Fusion of the joint gives a pain-free restricted, but powerful range of movements to the thumb and is suitable for manual workers. An excision arthroplasty will give greater movement at the base of the thumb but with a weaker grip. A silastic prosthesis will allow movement, relief of symptoms and a degree of strength but may be complicated by instability and fracture of the silastic prosthesis.
	B	**False**	
	C	**False**	
	D	**True**	
	E	**True**	
92	A	**True**	Morton's metatarsalgia is a painful, tender thickening of the common digital nerve usually between the third and fourth toes, or less commonly the second and third toes. The web space is painful on compression and sensory loss may be found within the web space and affected toes. The cause of the neuroma is unknown but may be due to repeated minor trauma. Excision of the neuroma usually relieves symptoms.
	B	**False**	
	C	**True**	
	D	**True**	
	E	**True**	

Questions (*Answers overleaf*)

93 Synovial chondromatosis has the following features

A The hip joint is most commonly affected
B Radiographs are sometimes diagnostic
C The occurence of multiple cartilaginous nodules within the villi of the synovial membrane
D Early cases may require arthroscopy for diagnosis
E Malignant change is frequent

94 In individuals with achondroplasia

A there will be proportionate short stature
B the limbs are short relative to the trunk
C impaired intelligence is common
D a large head with flattened nose is characteristic
E associated endocrine disturbances are invariable

95 Ganglia have the following characteristics

A They are cystic swellings associated with synovial joints or tendon sheaths
B They contain a clear jelly-like material
C Most frequently, they are found around the knee
D They are usually attached to skin
E They do not recur after excision

96 Chondrosarcomata

A may develop in the older age groups from a pre-existing condition such as Paget's disease or diaphyseal aclasis
B are rapidly fatal
C respond rapidly to chemotherapy
D metastasise early through the lymphatics
E show destruction of trabecular bone with irregular flecks of calcification and periosteal new bone formation on radiographs

Answers

93 A **False** Synovial chondromatosis is a disorder in which
B **True** multiple cartilage bodies develop on the synovial
C **True** membrane. Some may lose their attachment and
D **True** become loose bodies. The knee is most frequently
E **False** affected in young and middle-aged adults although the hip, elbows and wrist may also be affected. Radiographs will be normal unless the cartilaginous bodies calcify or ossify. Arthroscopy will demonstrate the multiple radiolucent granules within a joint and allow synovial biopsy. Severe cases may require synovectomy to clear the joint. While malignant change has been reported, it is rare.

94 A **False** Achondroplasia is the commonest form of dwarfism
B **True** and is associated with short limbs compared to the
C **False** trunk. The head is large with a flattened nose and
D **True** prominent forehead. Intelligence and sexual
E **False** function is normal. There is a familial tendency, though many cases are sporadic. No cause for the disorder is known.

95 A **True** A ganglion is a cystic swelling associated with a
B **True** synovial joint or tendon sheath. The majority occur
C **False** on the dorsal surface of the wrist, others at the foot
D **False** or knee. They consist of a dense fibrous tissue wall
E **False** and contain clear thick jelly-like material. Ganglia are not attached to skin but to the underlying joint or tendon sheath. They are usually tense but may be fluctuant. They may recur despite excision of the swelling.

96 A **True** Chondrosarcomata may arise de novo or secondary
B **False** to an underlying condition such as diaphyseal
C **False** aclasis, enchondromas, chondromas or Paget's
D **False** disease. In the latter group, age of presentation is
E **True** delayed, while the de novo tumours develop in the younger age groups. Most tumours are slow growing and metastasise late. Radiographs may show an expanding destructive lesion with flecks of calcification which may be invading soft tissue. The tumours are usually resistant to chemotherapy and require wide total excision or amputation of the limb.

Questions (*Answers overleaf*)

97 Ewing's tumours of bone
- **A** occur most commonly in the 30–60 year age group
- **B** are usually seen in the metaphyseal region of long bones
- **C** are resistant to treatment by chemotherapy
- **D** may present as a febrile illness and mimic acute osteomyelitis
- **E** have a tendency to involve several bones in many parts of the skeleton

98 In spinal tuberculosis
- **A** the infection develops in bone adjacent to a disc
- **B** new bone formation is minimal in active infection
- **C** radiographs usually show destruction of the body of a vertebra without involvement of the disc
- **D** an abscess in the lumbar region may track down the psoas sheath and produce a swelling in the groin
- **E** paraplegia may occur due to formation of an abscess within the spinal cord

99 Klippel-Feil syndrome
- **A** is a congenital condition in which there are developmental abnormalities of the cervical vertebrae including anomalies of segmentation
- **B** is associated with an abnormally long, stiff neck
- **C** frequently results in progressive neurological changes due to cord compression
- **D** is associated with Sprengel's shoulder
- **E** is usually associated with mental retardation

Answers

97 A **False** B **False** C **False** D **True** E **True**

Ewing's tumours occur typically in the 5–15 year age group. They often present as a febrile illness with pain and swelling in the diaphyseal area of the long bones, especially the tibia. Some patients may present with what appear to be multiple primary sites. Radiographs will show diffuse rarefaction towards the middle of the bone and over a period of time onion-skin layers may be seen produced by periosteal reaction. Histology shows a round cell tumour often in rosette formation, with areas of necrosis but without evidence of new bone formation. The tumours are sensitive to chemotherapy and radiotherapy.

98 A **True** B **True** C **False** D **True** E **True**

Spinal tuberculosis most frequently affects the lower thoracic vertebrae but may affect any part of the spine and at more than one level. The bacilli infect the marrow and destroy bone usually with very little reactive new bone formation. As the infection continues it affects the intervertebral disc and the adjacent vertebral body. Eventually there is collapse of the vertebrae to cause an angulatory deformity; a gibbus or kyphosis. With the development of further granulation tissue and debris, a cold abscess forms which may track from the lumbar region under the psoas sheath to beneath the inguinal ligament. An abscess may pass backwards into the spinal canal resulting in damage to the cord and eventual paraplegia.

99 A **True** B **False** C **False** D **True** E **False**

Klippel and Feil described a congenital abnormality of the neck in which the neck is short or absent and where there is marked limitation of movement. There may be other abnormalities including an elevated, small scapula (Sprengel's shoulder), facial asymmetry and scoliosis. Radiological examination may show failure of vertebral segmentation in the cervical and upper thoracic region, atlanto-axial fusion and spina bifida. Neurological complications may occur, but are uncommon. Usually the mental state is not affected.

Questions (*Answers overleaf*)

100 Poliomyelitis

A is a viral infection in which some of the anterior horn cells of the spinal cord are damaged either temporarily or permanently

B may result in leg length inequality when it affects one limb in infancy

C usually produces a short, rigid type of scoliosis

D may result in neuropathic ulcers under the foot which may be difficult to eradicate

E usually results in early degenerative arthritis of the knee when affecting muscles around the joint

101 Tuberculosis

A is caused by a Gram negative organism

B in Great Britain, is mainly the bovine type

C can arise de novo in bone

D usually arises in bone by haematogenous dissemination

E is more likely to affect synovial joints than the shafts of long bones

102 The following muscles in the hand are supplied by the ulnar nerve

A Abductor pollicis brevis

B The first dorsal interosseous muscle

C Adductor pollicis

D Abductor digiti minimi

E Opponens pollicis

Answers

100 A **True** B **True** C **False** D **False** E **False**

Poliomyelitis is a viral infection which causes a prodromal febrile illness associated with a varying degree of paralysis. It affects the anterior horn cells within the central nervous system in both the brain stem and spinal cord. The anterior horn cells may be totally destroyed, others are partially destroyed and contain Nissl granules on microscopy. There is no recovery of totally destroyed cells. The clinical picture is one of a lower motor neurone lesion varying in severity. It does not affect the sensory system. There may be leg-length inequality in children with long-standing disease in one limb. The scoliosis in poliomyelitis is usually a long c-shaped curve which is mobile. Osteoarthritis of joints in a limb affected by poliomyelitis is very uncommon unless operative treatment has been performed.

101 A **False** B **False** C **False** D **True** E **True**

Tuberculosis is caused by an acid-fast bacillus. The human type is now much commoner than the bovine, mainly due to pasteurisation of milk. Bone and joint infection is almost always secondary to a primary infection elsewhere. The organism spreads from its original focus via the blood stream to the skeletal system where it more frequently affects joints than shafts of long bones.

102 A **False** B **True** C **True** D **True** E **False**

The superficial branch of the ulnar nerve supplies the palmaris brevis muscle, part of the panniculus carnosus, and sensation to the ulnar one and a half fingers. The deep branch passes under the hook of the hamate between the origins of flexor and abductor digiti minimi which it supplies. It also supplies opponens digiti minimi, all the interossei, the ulnar two lumbrical muscles, and the two heads of adductor pollicis. The ulnar nerve therefore supplies all muscles in the hand excluding the muscles in the nemonic L.O.A.F. which are supplied by the median nerve;

L: Radial two lumbricals.
O: Opponens pollicis.
A: Abductor pollicis brevis.
F: Flexor pollicis brevis.

Questions (*Answers overleaf*)

103 In ulnar neuritis at the elbow

A the nerve may be compressed by a fibrous band as it passes under the lateral epicondyle
B the disorder may be a complication of an old un-united lateral condylar fracture
C the patient complains of paraesthesia over the ulnar border of the hand
D nerve conduction studies may confirm the diagnosis
E the nerve should be decompressed by division of the fibrous band or transposition to the anterior border of the medial epicondyle

104 In chronic osteomyelitis of the femur

A the sheath of new bone surrounding the original cortex is called the involucrum
B a loose dead infected segment of bone is called a sequela
C perforations within the bone through which pus escapes are called cloacae
D long standing skin sinuses may develop a carcinoma-in-situ
E the radiological picture may mimic osteosarcoma

Answers

103 A **False** B **True** C **True** D **True** E **True**

Ulnar neuritis most commonly occurs by compression at the elbow as the nerve passes under the medial epicondyle. The compression at the elbow may be caused by a fibrous band or by a valgus deformity caused by injury including an un-united fracture of the lateral condyle of the humerus or chronically dislocated radial head. It may also be caused by compression from rheumatoid tissue. Symptoms are pain and paraesthesia in the distribution of the ulnar nerve and weakness of the hand including the interossei and the muscles of the hypothenar eminence. Nerve conduction studies may show delayed conduction along the nerve. Treatment is aimed at releasing the nerve from its constriction by division of the band with or without transposition of the nerve.

104 A **True** B **False** C **True** D **True** E **True**

The sheath of new bone surrounding the original cortex is called the involucrum. Separated, necrotic and infected pieces of bone are referred to as sequestra and may be the cause of prolonged infection despite treatment with antibiotics. Perforations through the cortex, the cloacae, are caused by pus tracking under pressure to the surface and eventually through the skin. The epithelial lining of the skin sinuses over a long period of time may undergo malignant change to a squamous carcinoma-in-situ. Another complication is the deposition of amyloid in the liver, kidneys and spleen. Radiographs of chronic osteomyelitis and osteosarcoma may be very similar and include bone destruction, periosteal elevation and new bone formation.

Questions (*Answers overleaf*)

105 A 50 year old male presents with acute pain in his neck radiating over the shoulder, down the arm into the middle three fingers of his hand without any neurological abnormality on examination. Which of the following may aid diagnosis?

- **A** Cervical spine radiographs
- **B** Chest radiograph
- **C** A technetium 99m bone scan
- **D** An urgent radiculogram
- **E** A short course of steroids

106 In arthrogryposis multiplex congenita

- **A** the child is usually mentally retarded
- **B** there is a characteristic lack of skin creases and muscle contour
- **C** the joints of the upper limb are not affected
- **D** the disease is essentially a disorder of joint development
- **E** there is no sensory abnormality

107 A triple arthrodesis of the foot

- **A** includes the calcaneo-cuboid, talo-navicular and ankle joints
- **B** may be required for an ankle fracture which has developed incapacitating osteoarthritis
- **C** may be used to correct residual deformity of congenital talipes equinovarus including an inverted heel and adducted forefoot
- **D** in an adult, requires about 4 weeks in plaster before fusion occurs
- **E** is contra-indicated in women

Answers

105 A **True** B **True** C **True** D **False** E **False**

The history presented suggests a diagnosis of cervical spondylosis at about the level C6/C7. Less common causes to be excluded include tumours, especially secondary deposits and infection. Cervical spine and chest radiographs will help to differentiate several of the above causes. A negative bone scan will exclude a neoplastic deposit in the spine. A positive bone scan may show an occult secondary but may also show hot spots from degenerative changes in the neck. An urgent radiculogram is unlikely to be helpful unless gross neurological changes are present. Blood investigations should also be performed as well as a full careful general examination.

106 A **False** B **True** C **False** D **False** E **True**

Arthrogryposis multiplex congenita is a disease in which there are multiple joint deformities. It appears that the joints are not primarily involved but result from stiffness secondary to muscular fibrosis and wasting. The child may present with bilateral or unilateral club foot and rigid elbows and wrists. Any part of the body may be affected. There is a lack of skin creases around the joints. Sensation is normal and often the children have above average intelligence.

107 A **False** B **False** C **True** D **False** E **False**

A triple arthrodesis of the foot is an operation in which the subtalar joint, the calcaneo-cuboid and talo-navicular joints are denuded of articular cartilage to induce bony fusion. The procedure allows correction of both hindfoot and forefoot deformities by including in the operation suitable wedge excisions of bone. For example, for a heel in varus a wedge based laterally at the subtalar joint will allow the heel to be placed in a valgus position. For a successful operation the ankle joint should be normal otherwise pain will persist. Post-operatively, the foot is placed in the corrected position in a below-knee plaster. Sound fusion of the joints requires at least 12 weeks in plaster. The procedure should be delayed beyond the age of about 12 years to allow full growth of the foot and an optimal fusion rate, but the sex of the patient is irrelevant.

Questions (*Answers overleaf*)

108 Scheuermann's disease of the spine
- **A** is due to multifocal low grade infection
- **B** results in a thoracic lordosis in severe cases
- **C** presents with mild aching pain usually in the thoracic and upper lumbar spine
- **D** is associated with a spinal deformity which is fully correctable by lying flat
- **E** has radiological appearances which are characteristic

109 A 60 year old male complains of gradual stiffness and pain at the metatarsophalangeal joint of the great toe without angular deformity. The diagnosis of hallux rigidus is made
- **A** Gout should be excluded
- **B** A bone scan is essential to confirm diagnosis
- **C** Routine radiographs of the toe will show osteoarthritis
- **D** A history of injury may be significant
- **E** Blood cultures will be positive

110 Which of the following may be associated with leg length inequality?
- **A** Neurofibromatosis
- **B** Achondroplasia
- **C** Infantile septic arthritis of the hip
- **D** Marfan's syndrome
- **E** An arterio-venous fistula

Answers

108
A **False**
B **False**
C **True**
D **False**
E **True**

Scheuermann's disease is associated with a kyphosis in the thoracic spine. It may occasionally affect the upper lumbar spine. It usually occurs in the 10–20 year age group and may affect either sex. The cause of the disease is unknown but theories have included fragmentation of the vertebral ring epiphysis and persistance of the anterior vascular groove with consequent anterior vertebral wedging. The patient presents with an increasing cosmetic deformity or pain. The kyphosis is fixed and there may be tenderness over the spine. All blood investigations are normal, but radiological examination will show classical changes including irregularity of the intervertebral discs with fragmentation of the ring epiphyses.

109
A **True**
B **False**
C **True**
D **True**
E **False**

Gradual pain and stiffness at the metatarsophalangeal joint of the great toe without hallux valgus is not an uncommon disorder. It may be associated with chronic gout and a serum uric acid estimation may be valuable. Most cases appear to develop spontaneously whereas others are associated with trauma or rarely osteochondritis dissecans of the joint. A bone scan may be 'hot' but will not aid diagnosis. Blood cultures will not be helpful in the disease and infection would be excluded by the slow development of the disease.

110
A **True**
B **False**
C **True**
D **False**
E **True**

Unilateral congenital bone abnormalities including short femora, congenital dislocation of the hip, coxa vara and absence of the fibula or tibia may produce leg length inequality. Soft tissue abnormalities including neurofibromatosis and arterio-venous malformations should be considered. Abnormalities of bone growth include enchondromatosis, fibrous dysplasia, osteogenesis imperfecta and diaphyseal aclasis. Infantile infections including septic arthritis and osteomyelitis may produce severe inequality. Trauma, especially when the growth plate is damaged, may produce shortening, whereas a midshaft fracture may result in over-growth of bone. Neurological defects such as polio, cerebral palsy and spina bifida may result in leg length inequality.

Questions (*Answers overleaf*)

111 In regard to congenital metatarsus varus
- **A** the hindfoot is normal
- **B** the child may present as a case of in-toeing
- **C** early operative correction is essential
- **D** most cases resolve spontaneously
- **E** radiographs confirm that the deformity lies at the metatarsophalangeal joints

112 In an adolescent with peroneal spastic flat foot
- **A** there is a rigid varus deformity at the subtalar and midtarsal joints
- **B** there may be tarsal coalition
- **C** infection of the subtalar joint should be excluded
- **D** movements of the hindfoot, although restricted, are not painful
- **E** other signs of cerebral palsy will be present

113 Causes of a unilateral small foot include
- **A** diastematomyelia
- **B** congenital talipes equino-varus
- **C** diabetes
- **D** poliomyelitis
- **E** Morton's neuroma

Answers

111 A **True** B **True** C **False** D **True** E **False**

Congenital metatarsus varus is a common deformity in infants and children and should be differentiated from congenital talipes equinovarus. In the former, the deformity is at the tarso-metatarsal joints with the metatarsals adducted and in varus while the hindfoot is normal. Although severe deformity will be obvious at birth, milder cases may present with in-toeing when the child begins to walk. Most authorities state that the deformity, which is often bilateral, resolves spontaneously. Several corrective procedures are described in which a soft tissue release is performed at the metatarso-tarsal joints. Others describe reduction of the deformity by manipulation and serial corrective plasters.

112 A **False** B **True** C **True** D **False** E **False**

Peroneal spastic flat foot is a syndrome in which there is a rigid valgus deformity of the hindfoot and spasm of the peroneal muscles. It is usually painful and commonly occurs in adolescents. Many cases are associated with tarsal coalition, with a medial bony or cartilaginous bar between the talus and calcaneum or the calcaneum and navicular bones. Special radiographic views may be necessary to identify the bar. Rarer causes of the syndrome include hindfoot infection, osteoid osteoma and degenerative arthritis. Spasticity in this syndrome is related to the contracted peroneal muscles which produce the valgus deformity and not to spasticity associated with cerebral palsy.

113 A **True** B **True** C **False** D **True** E **False**

A unilateral small foot may be an indication of an underlying neurological defect including spina bifida or unilateral poliomyelitis. A diastematomyelia (a bony or fibrous band which splits the spinal cord in a saggital and longitudinal direction) should be excluded in radiographs of the spine. Investigations may require a myelogram to identify a fibrous band. Patients with rigid unilateral congenital talipes equino-varus also have a smaller foot on the affected side with a decreased calf bulk. This problem may be exacerbated by bony operations such as a wedge tarsectomy. Unilateral pes cavus will also cause a decrease in foot size.

Questions (*Answers overleaf*)

114 Duchenne muscular dystrophy

A is usually a sex-linked recessive disease affecting boys
B presents most frequently in the second decade
C is a self limiting disease in which life expectancy is normal
D affects the distal muscles more than the proximal in the early stages
E can be confirmed by muscle biopsy

115 In total hip replacement of the Charnley type

A the cement is polymethylmethacrylate
B high density polyethylene is used for the acetabular component
C rejection by the recipient is the commonest cause of loosening
D the diameter of the femoral head is 50 mm
E the cement may burn the skin if left in contact for too long

Answers

114 A **True**
B **False**
C **False**
D **False**
E **True**

Duchenne (pseudohypertrophic) muscular dystrophy has a sex-linked recessive inheritance, though it may occasionally be autosomal recessive. The disease usually presents before the fifth year of life, with a waddling gait and increasing muscular weakness affecting the proximal muscle groups more than then distal. A paradox to the muscle weakness is the increase in muscle bulk. Muscle biopsy and enzyme estimation of the serum creatine phosphokinase confirm diagnosis. The disease is progressive; most children being wheel-chair bound by their teens and dying from cardiac failure or respiratory infections in the second decade of life.

115 A **True**
B **True**
C **False**
D **False**
E **True**

The components of the Charnley total hip replacement consist of a high quality stainless steel femoral component with a head diameter of 22 mm. Various shapes of stem and neck are available for special circumstances. The acetabular component consists of high density polyethylene. The two components are fixed into place using polymethylmethacrylate cement which is made by mixing a liquid with a granular powder. An exothermic reaction occurs during polymerisation and hardening. Rejection of the components by the body is not a recognised complication of the procedure. Loosening is usually associated with mechanical breakdown between components or infection.

Questions (*Answers overleaf*)

116 A meningocele

- **A** is a cystic distension of the meninges, filled with cerebrospinal fluid which herniates through the space caused by failure of fusion of the vertebral arches
- **B** only occurs in the lumbar region of the spine
- **C** may be associated with a cutaneous hairy patch
- **D** is associated with serious lower limb neurological abnormalities
- **E** does not require treatment, even though the swelling may be large

117 In complete chronic rupture of the rotator cuff

- **A** pain is usually maximal in the arc of 60–120° of shoulder elevation
- **B** an arthrogram will confirm diagnosis
- **C** there is often a significant history of injury
- **D** pain rather than loss of function is the main indication for operative repair
- **E** routine radiographs of the shoulder are invariably normal

Answers

116
A **True**
B **False**
C **True**
D **False**
E **False**

Meningoceles are associated with spina bifida. They occur most frequently in the lumbo-sacral region although they may occur at any site along the spine. The meningocele consists of the meninges; dura mater, arachnoid mater and pia mater and is filled with cerebro-spinal fluid. The cystic swelling may be covered with skin and there may be an associated cutaneous hairy patch, naevus, lipoma or haemangioma. A cyst containing nerve tissue including nerve roots and a splayed-out spinal cord is called a myelomeningocele and may be open or covered by skin. A meningocele is not usually associated with a serious neurological deficit in the lower limbs, since the spinal cord and nerve roots are not affected. In myelomeningocele, serious neurological deficits may occur including bladder and bowel involvement. Closure of the meningocele is usually performed soon after birth to avoid complications of spontaneous rupture and infection.

117
A **False**
B **True**
C **False**
D **True**
E **False**

In a complete chronic rupture of the rotator cuff there may be a history of repetitive minor injury affecting the dominant upper limb. It usually occurs in the over fifties. The patient complains of shoulder pain with a subacromial tender area. The patient may 'hunch' his shoulder when starting abduction due to failure of the rotator cuff to initiate movement. Routine radiographs frequently show degenerative change especially at the acromio-clavicular and gleno-humeral joints. An arthrogram will show leakage of contrast from the shoulder joint into the subacromial bursa. Operative treatment is aimed primarily at the relief of pain rather than improved shoulder function.

Questions (*Answers overleaf*)

118 Calcification in the tendinous rotator cuff

- **A** is seen in the subacromial region on an antero-posterior radiograph of the shoulder
- **B** is frequently associated with a significant shoulder injury
- **C** can be an incidental finding
- **D** can present as acute pain with restriction of movements in the shoulder
- **E** is only seen after the 5th decade of life

119 Radiographic features of articular rheumatoid arthritis include

- **A** marked subchondral sclerosis
- **B** periarticular erosions in the early stages
- **C** absence of cyst formation
- **D** soft tissue swelling
- **E** destruction of the joint space

120 Concerning congenital subluxation of the wrist (Madelung's deformity)

- **A** The deformity consists of dorsal and lateral bowing of the distal radius with dorsal subluxation of the ulna
- **B** It is more common in boys
- **C** It is associated with premature fusion of the ulnar half of the distal radial epiphysis
- **D** It may be treated by shortening of the distal end of the ulna
- **E** It is usually unilateral

Answers

118 A **True**
B **False**
C **True**
D **True**
E **False**

Calcification within the rotator cuff may be an incidental finding on a radiograph. It may be associated with spontaneous acute intense pain over the deltoid with refusal to move the shoulder. The pain is due to the calcific deposit which causes an acute inflammatory reaction. It may occur in younger patients and because of pain, may require rapid treatment. In the early stages, an injection of hydrocortisone and local anaesthetic may relieve symptoms. After a few days, removal of the calcification may be necessary by operation.

119 A **False**
B **True**
C **False**
D **True**
E **True**

In the early stage of the disease, there are frequently no radiological changes in the joints apart from soft tissue swelling. Later peri-articular erosions develop especially in the phalanges. Generalised osteoporosis is a feature of later disease with loss of joint space and development of subchondral cysts which may be large. Osteophyte formation is often minimal unless changes of secondary osteoarthritis become superimposed on the rheumatoid features.

120 A **True**
B **False**
C **True**
D **True**
E **False**

Madelung's deformity is an abnormality of the distal end of the radius in which there is defective development of the ulnar side of the distal radial epiphysis, resulting in overgrowth of the lateral side of the radius and subsequent dorsal bowing. The ulna becomes dorsally subluxated. The deformity is often bilateral and more common in females. Clinically the hand and wrist are weak. Palmarflexion may be full, but dorsiflexion is restricted. Treatment in severe cases is by osteotomy of the distal radius to reduce palmar angulation. Sub-periosteal resection of the distal ulna also gives satisfactory results.

Questions (*Answers overleaf*)

121 Hyaline cartilage
- **A** obtains nutrition from synovial fluid
- **B** contains blood vessels originating from subchondral bone
- **C** shows many mitotic figures on routine histology
- **D** contains nerve fibres
- **E** is the main component of intervertebral discs

122 Horner's syndrome includes the following physical signs
- **A** A dilated pupil
- **B** Drooping of the eye lid
- **C** Exopthalmos
- **D** Lack of sweating over the forehead on the affected side
- **E** Weakness of the third cranial nerve

123 In Klumpke's obstetrical paralysis (lower plexus)
- **A** a frequent cause is forceful elevation and traction of the babies' arm away from the trunk
- **B** the shoulder muscles are invariably paralysed
- **C** the baby is likely to have Horner's syndrome
- **D** the intrinsic muscles of the hand are paralysed
- **E** separation of the upper humeral epiphysis may be seen on radiographs

Answers

121 A **True**
B **False**
C **False**
D **False**
E **False**

Hyaline cartilage, which covers the articular surface of synovial joints, contains no blood vessels, lymphatics or nerve fibres. It obtains its nutrition from synovial fluid produced by the lining membrane of the joint, the synovium. Movement of the joint aids movement of synovial fluid and indirectly the nutrition of articular cartilage. The chondrocytes within normal hyaline cartilage have a very poor mitotic activity although damage to the tissue results in clusters of chondrocytes which are believed to be due to replication of the cells. Intervertebral discs are mainly composed of fibrocartilage.

122 A **False**
B **True**
C **False**
D **True**
E **False**

A Horner's syndrome is due to paralysis of the sympathetic nerves from the first thoracic segments which pass to the superior cervical ganglion. The sympathetic nerve fibres pass via the internal carotid to the eye and associated structures. Interference with this supply results in a constricted pupil, with drooping of the upper lid and narrowing of the palpebral fissure. There is enopthalmos and absence of sweating over the forehead on the affected side. Eye movements are normal.

123 A **True**
B **False**
C **True**
D **True**
E **True**

Klumpke's obstetrical paralysis is caused by traction on an abducted arm resulting in stretching of the C8 and T1 nerve roots. This results in paralysis of the intrinsic muscles of the hand and the wrist and finger flexors. Damage to T1 close to the spinal cord may result in division of the sympathetics to the eye resulting in Horner's syndrome. In severe cases, radiographs of the shoulder may show an associated bony injury or dislocation of the shoulder.

Questions (*Answers overleaf*)

124 In marble bone disease (osteopetrosis)
- **A** the incidence is common
- **B** the cortices are thicker than normal
- **C** bone strength is increased
- **D** aplastic anaemia may develop in older patients
- **E** skull bone thickening may result in cranial nerve palsies

125 Metatarsalgia
- **A** is the symptom of pain under the metatarsal heads, usually made worse by weight bearing
- **B** frequently occurs in patients with rheumatoid disease
- **C** is associated in the older age groups with flattening or reversal of the transverse metatarsal arch
- **D** may be treated in patients with prominent metatarsal heads by displacement osteotomies through the necks of the metatarsals
- **E** invariably responds to a course of physiotherapy including faradic foot baths

126 Bipartite patellae
- **A** are only found in the skeletally immature
- **B** present with the smaller fragment usually at the upper, inner quadrant of the patella
- **C** are frequently bilateral
- **D** are probably anomalies of development
- **E** do not cause symptoms and are an incidental finding

Answers

124 A **False** B **True** C **False** D **True** E **True**

Marble bone disease (Albers-Schonberg) is a bone disorder in which awareness by students is out of proportion to its frequency. It is rare. Presumably the cause for this is the dramatic radiological appearance of increased bone density and obliteration of the medullary canal. Despite the increased thickness, the bones are soft and prone to pathological fracture. Complications also result from the thickening of bone around the cranial foramina producing nerve palsies and in long bones, to the loss of haemopoetic tissue in the medulla causing anaemia. There is a familial trend to the disorder with an autosomal recessive inheritance.

125 A **True** B **True** C **True** D **True** E **False**

Metatarsalgia is the symptom of pain under the heads of the metatarsals which may be caused by many foot disorders. Loss of muscle tone and ligament laxity with splaying of the foot results in extra strain on the metatarsal heads. This occurs in older patients, often in association with hallux valgus. Rheumatoid disease and diabetes are common causes of metatarsalgia. Morton's metatarsalgia (interdigital neuroma) and Freiberg's disease are less common causes. In the patients with splayed feet, physiotherapy and suitably padded insoles often relieve symptoms. However, it should be emphasised that metatarsalgia is a symptom and may be caused by disorders in which physiotherapy has little to offer. Osteotomies at the neck of the metatarsals may be used to relieve pressure as can excision of the heads of the metatarsals in suitable patients.

126 A **False** B **False** C **True** D **True** E **False**

The consensus view of bipartite patella is that it is a congenital anomaly. Most are bilateral. They are most frequently seen in the upper and outer quadrant of the patella and only occasionally at other sites. Bipartite patellae persist into adult life and may be the site of degenerative change in the adjacent articular cartilage. Occasionally it may be the site of painful chondromalacia patellae in adolescents. It is important to differentiate bipartite patella from a marginal fracture.

Questions (*Answers overleaf*)

127 In regard to deformities of the toes
- **A** Claw toes are hyperextended at the metacarpophalangeal joints and flexed at the interphalangeal joints
- **B** Painful claw toes may be treated by extensor tenotomy and proximal interphalangeal fusion
- **C** A hammer toe is hyperextended at the metatarsophalangeal joint, flexed at the proximal and extended at the distal interphalangeal joints
- **D** In hammer toes and claw toes, a frequent cause of pain is secondary osteoarthritis in the interphalangeal joints
- **E** An over-riding 5th toe may be congenital and familial

128 In scurvy
- **A** haemorrhages occur, causing subperiosteal haematomas around the metaphysis and growth plate in children
- **B** joint swellings are painless
- **C** radiological changes may be mistaken for osteomyelitis
- **D** there is an associated pyrexia
- **E** there is an inadequate intake of Vitamin C

129 A 3 year old child is seen in casualty. He is apyrexial but has multiple bruising around the buttocks, a painful swollen bruised knee and is undernourished. The parents deny a history of injury. The diferential diagnosis would include
- **A** Scurvy
- **B** Albright's syndrome
- **C** leukaemia
- **D** Perthe's disease
- **E** infective arthritis of the knee

Answers

127 A **True**
B **True**
C **True**
D **False**
E **True**

Claw toes are not uncommon and usually cause symptoms because of pressure on the skin over the dorsal surface of the proximal interphalangeal joints when wearing shoes. Treatment in resistant cases is by extensor tenotomy and proximal interphalangeal joint fusion. Hammer toes also cause symptoms from pressure on the skin of the dorsal surface of the proximal interphalangeal joints and at the tip of the toes when wearing shoes. Proximal interphalangeal joint fusion and extensor tenotomy at the metatarsophalangeal joint is performed in severe cases. Osteoarthritis in the affected joints in either deformity is not a significant cause of symptoms, even though degenerative changes may exist. Over-riding of the 5th toes, often bilateral, familial and congenital, is usually asymptomatic. In symptomatic cases, a soft tissue release to straighten the toe should improve symptoms.

128 A **True**
B **False**
C **True**
D **False**
E **True**

Scurvy is the clinical condition associated with a lack of Vitamin C (ascorbic acid). It results in haemorrhage into the gums, subcutaneous tissue and bone. The subperiosteal haemorrhages can be large, producing swollen, exquisitely tender limbs and swollen joints. Systemic effects are minimal, although the patient may appear malnourished. Radiological changes include periosteal elevation and when severe, displacement of the epiphysis. These changes may mimic osteomyelitis. Replacement of Vitamin C results in a rapid recovery.

129 A **True**
B **False**
C **True**
D **False**
E **False**

Scurvy may present with cutaneous bruising and haemorrhage into joints. The child would also have other manifestations including gingival haemorrhages. Acute leukaemia may also present with cutaneous haemorrhages and joint swellings. An infective arthritis is not likely since the child is apyrexial and bruising elsewhere would not be a feature. The battered baby syndrome is a strong possibility since there are signs of injury at several sites together with the fact that the baby is undernourished.

Questions (*Answers overleaf*)

130 Related to the above case history, which of the following would aid diagnosis of a battered baby?
- **A** Full blood count
- **B** High index of suspicion
- **C** Skeletal survey
- **D** A high erythrocyte sedimentation rate
- **E** Aspiration of the knee

131 Disc space infection of the spine, other than tubercle
- **A** presents with back pain and muscle spasm
- **B** will not show radiological abnormalities in the early stages
- **C** is most frequently a *Staphyloccus aureus* infection
- **D** is a known post-operative complication of a prostatectomy
- **E** requires early operative exploration

Answers

130 A **True**
B **True**
C **True**
D **False**
E **True**

A full blood count may show an iron deficiency anaemia due to repeated haemorrhage or nutritional deficit. A skeletal survey may show multiple fractures at various stages of healing suggesting repeated injury. An erythrocyte sedimentation rate would be normal. Aspiration of the knee may confirm a haemarthrosis due to trauma. A high index of suspicion and careful family history may aid diagnosis in all children with multiple sites of injury which cannot be explained by an underlying disease process.

131 A **True**
B **True**
C **True**
D **True**
E **False**

Spinal disc space infection, presenting with constant back pain, pyrexia and general malaise may occur at any age but is more common in the adult. It may occur spontaneously or be associated with distant sites of infection or operative procedures on the urinary tract including cystoscopy or prostatectomy. The lumbar region is most frequently involved. In the early stages, radiographs may be normal, though a technetium 99m bone scan may demonstrate a 'hot spot' at the site of the lesion. Later radiographs will show loss of disc space and lysis of bone of adjacent vertebrae. Needle biopsy of the lesion may confirm diagnosis and the culture usually grows *Staphylococcus aureus* and less frequently *E. coli*. Conservative treatment with appropriate antibiotic therapy and immobilisation of the spine in plaster is the treatment of choice. Serial erythrocyte sedimentation rates and radiographs are used to assess efficiency of treatment.

Questions (*Answers overleaf*)

132 A 60 year old male develops a slowly increasing weakness of the lower limbs with diminished sensation below the level of T10. He is admitted to hospital because of acute retention of urine. Which of the following should be carried out to obtain a diagnosis?

A Cystoscopy
B Chest radiographs
C Radiographs of the lumbo-sacral spine
D A myelogram
E Serum vitamin B_{12} estimation

133 Aneurysmal bone cysts

A only occur in the immature skeleton
B usually occur in the diaphyseal region of long bones
C show an eccentrically placed cystic lesion with expansion of the cortex on radiographs
D result in brisk haemorrhage when penetrated by a scalpel
E are treated by curettage and bone grafting with little risk of recurrence

134 Solitary (unicameral) bone cysts

A develop at any age
B may be a cause of pathological fracture
C start in the metaphysis and appear to migrate to the diaphysis with bone growth
D are solid, containing fibrous tissue
E do not result in expansion of the cortex

Answers

132 A **False** B **True** C **False** D **True** E **False**

The history of lower limb weakness and sensory loss with a sensory level, together with acute retention of urine is strongly suggestive of impending paraplegia due to pressure on the spinal cord. Apart from acute injury, malignant secondaries in the spine and infection are the likeliest causes. A chest radiograph may show a bronchial carcinoma or evidence of tubercle. Lumbo-sacral spine radiographs would probably be normal since the lesion is higher in the spine. Radiographs of the correct spinal level are necessary, otherwise important evidence may be missed. A myelogram will identify the level of obstruction. Other investigations would include a full blood count, erythrocyte sedimentation rate and special radiographic techniques in cases where a primary tumour is sought.

133 A **False** B **False** C **True** D **True** E **False**

Aneurysmal bone cysts may present at any age, but most commonly in the second and third decades. They are found in the metaphyseal region of long bones and also in the spine. The lesions are eccentrically placed and the cortex is often thinned and expanded. The cyst is multilocular and is filled with blood. Treatment is by curettage and obliteration of the cavity with bone chips. Recurrence is not uncommon, requiring further treatment. Inaccessible cysts including vertebral lesions may be treated by radiotherapy.

134 A **False** B **True** C **True** D **False** E **True**

Solitary bone cysts which occur in children, arise in the metaphyseal region and appear to move towards the diaphysis with bone growth. They may be asymptomatic or a site of pathological fracture. They do not expand the cortex, but fill the diameter of the bone. The unilocular cysts contains fluid, which is normally yellow in colour, but may be blood stained if subject to recent trauma. The cysts may be treated by removing the thin lining and filling the cavity with bone chips. Recurrence of the cyst may occur especially in young children requiring further grafting.

Questions (*Answers overleaf*)

135 Concerning bone growth in the immature skeleton

A Widening of a long bone is due to periosteal bone formation

B Lengthening of a bone occurs with new bone formation on the diaphyseal side of the growth plates

C Injury to the growth plate invariably results in an increase in bone length

D Excess thyroid hormone results in decreased bone growth, with bone age less than chronological age

E Abnormal muscle activity in disorders such as polio affect bone growth

136 Regarding osteogenesis imperfecta

A There is no evidence of a hereditary disorder

B All patients present within the first year of life

C Blood biochemistry shows a low serum calcium

D Fractures often fail to heal

E Some patients have blue sclerae

Answers

135 A **True**
B **True**
C **False**
D **False**
E **True**

Bone growth in the immature skeleton occurs in both a longitudinal direction and by widening of the bone. Longitudinal growth occurs at the growth plates at the ends of the bone. Here cartilage cells proliferate on the diaphyseal side which calcify and then ossify to form new bone (enchondral ossification). Increased width of the bone occurs by periosteal cellular proliferation and ossification. Factors affecting bone growth include hormonal factors including thyroxine and growth hormone and also local factors such as muscle activity and injury near or at the growth plate. Direct injury to the growth plate may result in premature fusion resulting in growth arrest, whereas increased blood supply to an adjacent fracture may stimulate bone growth.

136 A **False**
B **False**
C **False**
D **False**
E **True**

Osteogenesis imperfecta is a hereditary disease in which there is abnormal fragility or brittleness of bones. While some offspring develop fractures in utero and may be still-born, less severe forms manifest themselves in the first year of life or as the child becomes older. Despite the frequency of fracture, they unite in the usual time but often with deformity. Less severely affected children may have blue sclerae due to thinning of the sclerae allowing the colour of the choroid to show through. Blood biochemistry is usually normal, although with recent fractures, the alkaline phosphatase may be raised.

Questions (*Answers overleaf*)

137 In cerebral palsy

- **A** marked adduction contracture of the hips may be treated by adductor tenotomy and anterior obturator neurectomy
- **B** subluxed or dislocated hips require treatment in young children
- **C** an equinus deformity of the ankle may be treated by elongation of the tendo-achillis
- **D** bracing and splintage to reduce deformity has little value
- **E** results of correct treatment are related to the intelligence of the patient

138 Freiberg's disease

- **A** may be an incidental finding on radiographs of the foot
- **B** most commonly affects the metatarsal of the fourth toe
- **C** is usually bilateral
- **D** occurs most commonly in mature, overweight females
- **E** invariably requires excision of the head of the metatarsal as a primary procedure

Answers

137 A **True**
B **True**
C **True**
D **False**
E **True**

The aim of treatment in cerebral palsy is to reduce deformity and improve function. In the early stages of deformity, passive stretching and serial splintage may prevent serious contractures and obviate the need for surgery. In more severe deformities surgery may be necessary for correction and to aid mobilisation. Marked adduction contracture of the hips from weak abductors and overactive adductors may require adductor tenotomy and anterior obturator neurectomy to improve gait and also prevent subluxation of the hips. Subluxed or dislocated hips should be treated, again to improve mobility and also to prevent painful secondary osteoarthritis. A tight tendo-achillis may be lengthened to correct a fixed equinus deformity of the ankle. Overall, the results of correct treatment in patients with cerebral palsy are related to intelligence since the more intelligent the patient, the more likely he is to utilise improvement of the deformities.

138 A **True**
B **False**
C **False**
D **False**
E **False**

Freiberg's disease (osteochondritis of the metatarsal head), while occasionally being an incidental radiological finding, usually presents in childhood with swelling and pain in the second or third metatarsophalangeal joint. While its initial description was that of an osteochondritis, several authorities believe that it is caused by injury and sometimes occurs in a toe that is longer than normal. Most cases are unilateral. Initial treatment includes a below-knee plaster or an injection of hydrocortisone into the joint. With development of secondary osteoarthritis, excision of the metatarsal head has been suggested for persistent symptoms.

Questions (*Answers overleaf*)

139 Concerning the anatomy of the spine and spinal cord in the adult

A The distal end of the spinal cord lies at the level of the second sacral vertebra
B Cerebro-spinal fluid lies between the dura and arachnoid mater
C The cauda equina consists of the lower segments of the spinal cord and the lumbar and sacral nerve roots
D Mixed spinal nerves originate at the intervertebral foramina when posterior and anterior nerve roots join
E The immediate covering of the spinal cord is the dura mater

140 In a patient with sciatica, which of the following are correct?

A Decreased sensation over the outer aspect of the calf suggests an S1 nerve root lesion
B An absent ankle jerk suggests an L5 nerve root lesion
C Decreased sensation over the lateral aspect of the sole of the foot suggests an S1 nerve root lesion
D Weakness of the extensor hallucis longus suggests an L5 nerve root lesion
E Weakness of the gluteus maximus suggests an S1 nerve root lesion

141 The following are associated with Erb's Palsy

A A lesion of the upper trunk of the brachial plexus
B Excessive downward traction on the arm against a lateral traction force on the neck
C The shoulder lies internally rotated and the forearm pronated
D The small muscles of the hand are not affected
E The nerve roots of C6 and C7 are involved

Answers

139 A **False** B **False** C **False** D **True** E **False**

The spinal cord, covered by three layers, the dura, arachnoid and pia mater, ends at the conus medullaris opposite the first or second lumbar vertebrae. The dura mater extends to about the level of the second sacral vertebra. The pia mater covers the spinal cord and passes as the filum terminale to the second sacral vertebra. Between the dura and the pia lies the arachnoid mater and between the latter two layers, cerebro-spinal fluid. Between the level of the first or second lumbar vertebrae and the sacrum lies the cauda equina containing nerve roots, but no cord. The posterior and anterior nerve roots join at the intervertebral foramina to form mixed spinal nerves.

140 A **False** B **False** C **True** D **True** E **True**

A disc prolapse producing sciatica may produce objective signs of motor or a sensory deficit. Pressure on the L5 nerve root will produce weakness of the dorsiflexors of the toes especially the great toe and dorsiflexion of the ankle. Sensory changes may result in diminished sensation over the lateral border of the calf and dorsum of the foot. An S1 nerve root lesion will produce weakness of gluteus maximus and the foot plantarflexors together with loss of sensation over the lateral border of the sole of the foot and a decreased ankle jerk (ankle jerk S1, S2 nerve roots).

141 A **True** B **True** C **True** D **True** E **False**

Erb's palsy is caused by traction on the arm against a neck flexed to the opposite side. The upper trunk of the brachial plexus is stretched and torn. This may result in permanent paralysis or recovery. The shoulder girdle muscles innervated by C5 and C6 nerve roots are affected together with elbow flexors and brachio-radialis. Unopposed muscle activity results in the typical deformity of internal rotation of the shoulder and a pronated forearm.

Questions (*Answers overleaf*)

142 Sciatica from an acute prolapsed intervertebral disc
- **A** most commonly occurs in the over 40 year age group
- **B** rarely occurs in women
- **C** is usually caused by a sudden twisting injury of the spine
- **D** most commonly involves the second lumbar nerve root
- **E** requires urgent operative treatment to relieve pain

143 In degenerative spinal stenosis, with neurogenic claudication
- **A** peripheral pulses are invariably absent
- **B** pain, usually low back and radiating to the lower limbs, is made worse by walking
- **C** the patient is usually under 40 years
- **D** routine radiographs of the spine frequently show bony abnormalities
- **E** an acute prolapsed intervertebral disc is the most frequent treatable cause

144 Secondary affects of untreated chronic gout include
- **A** renal stones
- **B** chronic renal failure
- **C** soft tissue swellings over bony prominences
- **D** ulnar drift of the fingers at the metacarpo-phalangeal joints
- **E** optic atrophy

Answers

142 A **False** B **False** C **False** D **False** E **False**

Acute prolapsed intervertebral discs occur most frequently in the under 40 year age group in both men and women. There appears to be an underlying defect within the disc which predisposes to rupture, since the vast majority of patients deny any specific serious history of injury. The most frequent levels involved are the L5 and S1 nerve roots. Treatment is initially conservative with bed rest to relieve pain. Operative treatment is reserved for patients who fail to respond to conservative measures and those with a serious neurological deficit including acute urinary retention or a foot drop.

143 A **False** B **True** C **False** D **True** E **False**

Spinal stenosis, most commonly occuring in males over the age of 40 years, frequently presents with a history of increasing pain and paraesthesiae in the buttocks and thighs with walking, which is relieved by sitting forward or lying flat. The most common cause is degenerative disease within the spinal canal or intervertebral foramen which encroach on the nerve roots and spinal cord. While bulging of degenerate discs may add to the congestion, acute disc prolapse is not a recognised factor in degenerative spinal stenosis. Routine radiographs usually show osteophytic swellings around the facet joints, loss of disc spaces and syndesmophytes between vertebrae. Disturbances in the distal vascular tree in patients with spinal stenosis are coincidental but may cause diagnostic problems, especially if they produce vascular claudication.

144 A **True** B **True** C **True** D **False** E **False**

Chronic gout leads to destructive changes and secondary osteoarthritis within the joints involved, including the great toe metacarpophalangeal joints. Gouty tophi may develop in the soft tissue, especially the pinna of the ear and bony prominences including elbow, hands and feet. Deposition of urate crystals in the kidneys may result in chronic renal failure and renal stones. It should be observed, however, that not all patients with uric acid stones have hyperuricaemia or gout.

Questions (*Answers overleaf*)

145 Gout

A is caused by an abnormality of purine metabolism, in the primary type
B may be the first indication of chronic renal disease
C inevitably occurs in all patients with hyperuricaemia
D may be precipitated in a previously normal patient who takes a course of asprin
E only occurs in patients with a high alcohol intake

146 Extra-articular manifestations of rheumatoid arthritis include

A rheumatoid nodules typically seen on the flexor surfaces of joints
B nail bed or nail fold haemorrhages
C a macrocytic anaemia
D splenomegaly and leucopenia
E a pericarditis which is often asymptomatic

Answers

145 A **True** B **True** C **False** D **True** E **False**

Gout is a disorder in which precipitated crystals of monosodium urate within a joint produce an intense inflammatory reaction. Primary gout is caused by an abnormality of purine metabolism resulting in hyper-uricaemia. Secondary gout caused by an increased breakdown of purine may be seen in myeloproliferative and malignant disease. Hyper-uricaemia may also be caused by decreased excretion of uric acid following drug therapy or in chronic renal disease. Not all patients with hyper-uricaemia develop gout, but as the urate levels increase probability of crystal deposition becomes more likely. Other factors associated with crystal deposition include trauma and a sudden elevation of urate level.

146 A **False** B **True** C **False** D **True** E **True**

Patients with moderate to severe rheumatoid disease frequently have a normocytic normochromic anaemia. Rheumatoid nodules, frequently found in the subcutaneous tissues over the extensor surfaces of joints, are said to be an adverse prognostic factor. A vasculitis may develop affecting small size vessels to produce small infarcts and haemorrhages, peripheral neuropathy and ulcers. Splenomegaly, leucopaenia and rheumatoid arthritis is described as Felty's syndrome. Eye disorders include scleritis and kerato-conjunctivitis sicca. Respiratory diseases include pleural effusions and interstitial fibrosis. Pericarditis, usually asymptomatic, is a further extra-articular manifestation. Renal problems including glomerulitis and the nephrotic syndrome from amyloid are uncommon extra-articular manifestations of rheumatoid disease.

Questions (*Answers overleaf*)

147 In the treatment of osteoarthritis of the knee

A physiotherapy has no value even in mild cases
B a high tibial osteotomy is indicated when it affects mainly the medial compartment providing deformity is not severe
C knee arthrodesis is the treatment of choice in bilateral cases
D total knee replacement is the treatment of choice in the under 40 year age group
E a high tibial osteotomy will increase the range of movements in a stiff knee joint

148 Deformities following poliomyelitis include

A a severe fixed flexion deformity of the elbow
B a fixed flexion deformity of the knee
C an equinus deformity of the ankle
D limb lengthening on the affected side in unilateral diseases
E a scoliosis

149 Perthe's disease

A usually presents with a painful limp
B may present with pain in the knee
C frequently presents with limitation of all hip movements, especially internal rotation and abduction
D is associated with an intermittent pyrexia in the early stages
E may occasionally be an incidental finding on radiographs taken for an unrelated problem

Answers

147 A **False** B **True** C **False** D **False** E **False**

Treatment of osteoarthritis of the knee depends on the severity of the disease. In mild cases, physiotherapy including isometric quadriceps exercises and heat therapy often reduce symptoms. In more severe cases, especially in patients with only the medial compartment involved, an osteotomy to realign the knee and transfer load to the less involved side usually improves symptoms. A high tibial osteotomy for medial compartment osteoarthritis with a varus deformity will relieve pain but requires a good range of movements preoperatively. Bilateral disease is a strong indication for total joint replacement since function will be much better than arthrodesis.

148 A **False** B **True** C **True** D **False** E **True**

Deformities associated with poliomyelitis develop by a combination of muscle paralysis, the effects of gravity and unopposed muscle activity. In children, paralysed muscle and tendons become longer whereas active muscles tend to grow less due to absence of stretch reflexes from the weak or absent antagonists. At the ankle, equinus of the ankle occurs due to active calf muscles and weak dorsiflexors. Flexion deformity at the elbow is not usually severe despite a weak triceps muscle because gravity tends to extend the elbow. At the knee, a flexion deformity is common due to unopposed action of the hamstring muscles. A scoliotic paralytic curve is common and while mobile in the early stages, becomes a long fixed curve. Limb shortening is frequent in the affected limb.

149 A **True** B **True** C **True** D **False** E **True**

A frequent presentation of Perthe's disease is an intermittent limp with pain in the groin, anterior thigh or knee. Rarely, marked changes may be found on a radiograph without symptoms referrable to the hip joint. Restriction of movement, especially internal rotation and abduction are the chief presenting signs. The disease is not associated with a pyrexia or other systemic manifestation. Biochemical investigations are normal.

Questions (*Answers overleaf*)

150 Concerning the anatomical snuff box at the wrist

A The abductor pollicis brevis and extensor pollicis brevis form one boundary
B Extensor pollicis longus forms a second boundary
C The radial nerve can be palpated beneath extensor pollicis longus
D The radial artery can be palpated on the floor of the triangle
E The floor of the snuff box consists only of the radial styloid

151 In radial club hand (congenital absence of the radius)

A about half the patients have bilateral deformity
B the wrist is ulnar deviated at right angles to the forearm
C without treatment, function of the upper limb is poor
D there may be an associated absence or hypoplasia of the thumb
E mental retardation is very common

152 The pathological features of articular rheumatoid arthritis include

A proliferation of the synovial cells to produce a thick pannus
B enzyme production within articular cartilage which results in cartilage destruction
C increased bone formation around an affected joint
D a synovial fluid containing proteolytic enzymes
E contracture of ligaments resulting in lax joints

Answers

150 A **False**
B **True**
C **False**
D **True**
E **False**

The 'snuff box' at the wrist lies between the tendons of abductor pollicis longus and extensor pollicis brevis and the tendon of extensor pollicis longus. The cutaneous branches of the radial nerve can be palpated as they run over the extensor pollicis longus tendon across the snuff box. The bony floor consists of the radial styloid, scaphoid, trapezium and the base of the thumb metacarpal. Overlying the floor and beneath the tendons is the radial artery.

151 A **True**
B **False**
C **False**
D **True**
E **False**

Radial club hand is a deformity in which the radius is absent or hypoplastic and the wrist is deviated radially, often at right angles to the forearm. The thumb and radial carpal bones may be hypoplastic or absent. About half the children have a bilateral deformity and there may be other associated congenital abnormalities. Despite the deformity, function is often good. Operative treatment is aimed at realigning the wrist with the forearm preferably during the first year of life.

152 A **True**
B **False**
C **False**
D **True**
E **False**

In a synovial joint affected by rheumatoid arthritis, the essential feature is that the synovial lining becomes oedematous, proliferative and highly vascular. It is infiltrated with plasma cells and immune complexes. There is increased vascular permeability with release of enzymes including elastase, collagenase and cathepsins which damage the articular cartilage. This pannus grows over and into the cartilage which becomes fragmented and damaged. The ligaments and capsule stretch due to joint effusions and direct involvement by rheumatoid tissue and the bone surrounding the joint becomes porotic due to disuse and the effect of prostaglandins and other enzymes.

Questions (*Answers overleaf*)

153 In the anatomy of the foot and ankle
- **A** the tibialis posterior tendon passes anterior to the medial malleolus
- **B** peroneus brevis inserts into the base of the great toe metatarsal
- **C** the skin of the dorsum of the foot is supplied by the S2 dermatome
- **D** the talus is devoid of tendinous insertions
- **E** the lateral plantar nerve has a corresponding distribution of muscle innervation in the foot as the median nerve in the hand

154 Bow legs (genu varum) in a child of 2 years
- **A** is a common normal variant
- **B** are likely to progress into adulthood
- **C** are often a cause of delayed walking
- **D** may be due to an underlying pathological bone problem
- **E** require urgent treatment by stapling of the medial part of the upper tibial epiphysis

155 The following are causes of a thoracic kyphosis
- **A** Tuberculosis
- **B** Osteoporosis
- **C** Ankylosing spondylitis
- **D** A spondylolisthesis at L5–S1
- **E** Scheuermann's disease

Answers

153 A **False**
B **False**
C **False**
D **True**
E **False**

The structures passing behind the lateral malleolus of the ankle are the peroneus longus and brevis, with the latter inserting into the base of the 5th metatarsal. On the medial side of the foot, the tibialis posterior passes beneath and behind the medial malleolus to the navicular bone. The talus has neither insertions or origins of any muscle attached to it. The segmental sensory innervation of the dorsum of the foot is the fifth lumbar to the medial side of the foot and the first sacral to the lateral side. The lateral plantar nerve supplies the abductor digiti minimi, flexor digiti minimi, adductor hallucis, interossei and lateral lumbricals. The distribution is similar to the ulnar nerve in the hand.

154 A **True**
B **False**
C **False**
D **True**
E **False**

Mild bow legs caused by an increased bilateral lateral curvature of either the femur or tibia is a frequent developmental finding in the first two to three years of life. This type of deformity corrects itself with increasing age and does not result in delayed walking. Rarely bow legs may be a manifestation of underlying disease such as rickets, bone dysplasia and rarely Blount's disease, a disorder of growth of the medial tibial epiphysis.

155 A **True**
B **True**
C **True**
D **False**
E **True**

A kyphosis is a curvature of the spine, convex posteriorly which is greater than normal. It may occur as a postural abnormality in young girls which resolves when lying flat. A structural kyphosis may be caused by congenital bone abnormalities of the spine or Scheuermann's disease in adolescents. In young adults, ankylosing spondylitis may be the underlying cause and in the elderly, osteoporosis (Dowager's hump). Tuberculosis with anterior wedging between adjacent vertebrae produces a kyphosis, which is also called a 'gibbus'.

Questions (*Answers overleaf*)

156 Pseudogout

- **A** is caused by deposition of calcium pyrophosphate crystals within synovial joints
- **B** is common in children
- **C** may cause calcification of the knee menisci
- **D** in the acute stage, may be treated by irrigation of the joint with saline
- **E** may be prevented by long term allopurinol

157 Generalised joint laxity is associated with the following conditions

- **A** Rheumatoid arthritis
- **B** Myositis ossificans progressiva
- **C** Ehlers-Danlos syndrome
- **D** Arthrogryposis multiplex
- **E** Osteoarthritis

158 Idiopathic adolescent scoliosis

- **A** occurs most commonly in boys
- **B** most frequently affects the lumbar spine
- **C** is associated with a posterior rib prominence on the convex side of a thoracic curve
- **D** usually progresses rapidly after skeletal maturity
- **E** normally presents with pain

Answers

156 A **True** B **False** C **True** D **True** E **False**

Chondrocalcinosis (pseudogout) is caused by deposition of calcium pyrophosphate crystals within synovial joints. Large joints, especially the knee, are usually involved with acute severe pain and swelling, low-grade pyrexia and a warm joint. The symptoms tend to settle spontaneously, but arthroscopic saline irrigation of large joints often relieves pain more rapidly. Diagnosis is by confirmation of calcium pyrophosphate crystals in the synovial fluid using polarised microscopy and by calcification within the menisci and articular cartilage. The disease tends to occur in the older age groups and is controlled by anti-inflammatory agents including indomethacin.

157 A **False** B **False** C **True** D **False** E **False**

Generalised joint laxity may be a normal variant and related to age and race. Children tend to have more lax joints than adults and certain races, Asians for example, are more lax than Europeans. Clinical disorders associated with joint laxity include Ehlers-Danlos syndrome and Marfan's syndrome. Patients with rheumatoid arthritis and ligamentous damage due to trauma, the knee for example, have localised joint laxity. Patients with arthrogryposis, myositis ossificans progressiva and osteoarthritis have stiff joints.

158 A **False** B **False** C **True** D **False** E **False**

Idiopathic adolescent scoliosis is more frequently seen in girls than boys. It is most common in the thoracic region with the convexity to the right. There is a rotational deformity of the vertebrae resulting in a rib prominence in the thoracic region on the convex side of the scoliosis. Curve progression tends to be accelerated during the adolescent growth spurt whereas after skeletal maturity, progression is minimal. The presenting feature is usually the cosmetic defect of spinal curvature or rib prominence. Pain is not a significant feature in idiopathic adolescent scoliosis.

Questions (*Answers overleaf*)

159 Coccydynia

- **A** most commonly occurs in men
- **B** may follow a fracture of the coccyx
- **C** may be caused by a tumour of the sacro-coccygeal region
- **D** can be treated by an injection of local anaesthetic and hydrocortisone in post- traumatic cases
- **E** may be confused with referred pain from compression of the cauda equina by a prolapsed intervertebral disc

160 Concerning the following eponyms

- **A** Shenton's line is broken in congenital dislocation of the hip
- **B** Heberden's nodes are osteophytic swellings of the proximal interphalangeal joints
- **C** Ranvier's nodes are the synapses between the sensory and motor fibres of the reflex arc
- **D** Trethowan's sign is positive in a slipped upper femoral epiphysis
- **E** Schmorl's nodes are probably due to rupture of the intervertebral disc through the vertebral end plate

Answers

159 A **False** B **True** C **True** D **True** E **True**

Coccydynia is the term describing pain around the coccygeal region of the spine. It occurs most commonly in women and may result from a fracture of the coccyx, childbirth, a tumour, infection or arthritis of the sacro-coccygeal joint. A differential diagnosis is compression of the cauda equina within the spinal canal producing referred pain to the coccyx. Radiographs and a bone scan together with blood investigation will exclude more sinister causes of coccydynia and in the post-traumatic cases, short wave diathermy, hydrocortisone injection or manipulation under anaesthetic may be helpful. Excision of the coccyx is hardly ever indicated.

160 A **True** B **False** C **False** D **True** E **True**

Shenton's line lies along the upper border of the obturator foramen and continues laterally and inferiorly along the undersurface of the femoral neck. It is broken in congenital dislocation of the hip. Heberden's nodes are found in the terminal interphalangeal joints of the fingers and are osteophytic outgrowths. Ranvier's nodes are the constrictions seen in the axis cylinders of a myelinated nerve fibre. In slipped upper femoral epiphysis, a line drawn along the upper border of the neck passes above the head rather than through it (Trethowan's sign). Schmorl's nodes are seen in the bodies of vertebrae and are believed to be due to rupture of the intervertebral disc through the vertebral end plate.

Questions (*Answers overleaf*)

161 In the thoracic outlet syndrome

A the middle trunk of the brachial plexus is usually compressed

B the patient often complains of pain and paraesthesia along the medial aspect of the forearm and skin over the ring and little fingers

C compression may be caused by a cervical rib or fibrous band

D an audible bruit may be heard from the subclavian artery in the supraclavicular fossa

E vascular problems due to constriction of the brachial artery may produce attacks of dusky cyanosis in the fingers

162 In a patient suspected of a pulmonary embolus following a total hip replacement

A one or other of the lower limbs will invariably be swollen and oedematous

B cardiac arrest may be the first indication of the complication

C sudden chest pain with dyspnoea and tachycardia are frequent presenting symptoms

D the venous thrombosis is invariably present in the operated limb

E anticoagulant therapy is contraindicated in confirmed cases because of wound complications

Answers

161 A **False** B **True** C **True** D **True** E **False**

The thoracic outlet syndrome is due to compression of the brachial plexus, especially the lower trunk, and the subclavian artery as they pass over the first rib. The pathogenesis of the syndrome is complex but is related to abnormalities such as a cervical rib or fibrous band, a tight scalenus medius muscle or anomalies of the first rib. The patient frequently complains of paraesthesia along the medial border of the forearm and little and ring fingers, the distribution of the sensory component of the lower brachial trunk. There may be motor weakness affecting the small muscles of the hand. Vascular problems, which are uncommon, may include emboli or attacks of dusky cyanosis due to constriction of the subclavian artery at the thoracic outlet. Locally, there may be increased pulsations of the subclavian artery associated with a palpable bruit due to narrowing of the artery.

162 A **False** B **True** C **True** D **False** E **False**

Pulmonary embolus is a recognised complication of total hip replacement. At worst, it may result in sudden death or more frequently with sudden, sharp chest pain, breathlessness and haemoptysis. The venous thrombosis may occur in either the operated or unoperated limb and may not be associated with calf pain, swelling and a positive Homan's sign. In other words there may be no physical signs of thrombosis in the leg. Treatment by anticoagulants is the treatment of choice despite the recent operation providing the anticoagulation can be carefully controlled.

Questions (*Answers overleaf*)

163 Wry neck (torticollis)
- **A** when caused by a tight sternomastoid muscle results in lateral flexion of the head to the opposite side and rotation of the head to the same side
- **B** may be caused by congenital bony abnormalities of the cervical spine
- **C** can be a sign of a unifacetal dislocation of the cervical spine
- **D** may indicate an infection in the cervical spine
- **E** is associated with facial asymmetry in patients with infantile torticollis

164 In regard to arthrodesis of the shoulder
- **A** movement at the scapulo-thoracic joint is essential for a good functional result
- **B** a paralysed deltoid muscle is a contraindication to the operation
- **C** the arm should be fixed in the neutral position of rotation
- **D** good elbow function is a prerequisite of a successful shoulder arthrodesis
- **E** the patient is unlikely to be able to bring his hand to his mouth despite arthrodesis in a good position and good muscle control

Answers

163 A **False** B **True** C **True** D **True** E **True**

Wry-neck or torticollis is the description applied to the abnormality in which the head and neck are rotated and flexed to one side. The deformity may present in infants due to tightness of the sternomastoid muscle from fibrosis secondary to infarction or bleeding into the muscle. The tight sternomastoid results in lateral flexion of the neck to its own side and rotation of the neck to the opposite side. Prolonged torticollis in infants may result in facial asymmetry with the face on the affected side becoming longer. Other causes of torticollis are congenital bony abnormalities including the Klippel-Feil syndrome and cervical scoliosis. In a unifacetal dislocation of the cervical spine, there may be a torticollis which is painful especially when attempts are made to straighten the neck. An acute pyogenic infection in the cervical region including bone and soft tissue may present with a painful acute torticollis which is relieved by appropriate treatment.

164 A **True** B **False** C **False** D **True** E **False**

Arthrodesis of the shoulder may be indicated in severe glenohumeral joint destruction due to infection, trauma and arthritis. It may also be necessary in muscle paralysis. To be successful, it requires good movement and muscle function at the scapulo-thoracic joint and in the distal joints. Deltoid paralysis is not a contraindication to opeation since the muscle is no longer necessary after arthrodesis. The optimal position of arthrodesis is about 40° of abduction, 20° of forward flexion and 25° of internal rotation. A trial in a plaster with the shoulder held in the anticipated arthrodesed position is advisable to predict functional activity after operation. The patient should be able to place his hand into his pocket and reach his mouth with his hand.

Questions (*Answers overleaf*)

165 In deformities of the elbow

- **A** cubitus valgus may be caused by malunion of a fracture of the lateral condyle
- **B** malunion of a supracondylar fracture is more likely to result in valgus deformity than varus
- **C** an unreduced dislocation of the radial head may result in cubitus valgus in the long term
- **D** following a supracondylar fracture in children, premature fusion of the capitellar growth plate is a frequent cause of a valgus deformity
- **E** infection of the lateral condyle of the humerus in children may result in a cubitus varus deformity

166 Ingrowing toe nails

- **A** most frequently affect the great toe
- **B** are caused by pressure of the nail on the skin of the nail fold together with secondary infection
- **C** may require permanent ablation of the nail bed in resistant cases
- **D** when they become chronic, develop nail thickening resulting in onychogryphosis
- **E** frequently present with pain

167 Trendelenburg's test

- **A** is a test for a fixed flexion deformity of the hip joint
- **B** tests the stability of the pelvis on the femur
- **C** depends on the efficient function of the hip abductors
- **D** is best performed with the patient lying flat
- **E** is positive when the patient stands on one leg and the opposite iliac crest dips lower than the one on which the patient is standing

Answers

165 A **True** B **False** C **True** D **False** E **False**

In the normal elbow, the angle between the humerus and forearm with the elbow extended is 0° or with slight valgus up to 10°. An increase in this angle, the carrying angle, may be due to malunion of a lateral condylar fracture, excision of the radial head, and more rarely to a supracondylar fracture or an epiphyseal injury from trauma or infection. Cubitus varus deformity, in which the forearm is adducted on the humerus, is most frequently caused by malunion of a supra-condylar fracture and more rarely by an epiphyseal injury to the elbow due to infection or trauma.

166 A **True** B **True** C **True** D **False** E **True**

Ingrowing toe nails are common and cause pain, especially by pressure of a shoe on the toe nail. They are caused by the nail pushing into the skin of the nail fold with subsequent infection and pain. The great toe is most frequently affected, usually the lateral side, though some may affect both nails folds. Treatment is conservative initially, allowing the nail to grow out of the nail fold. Chronic cases may be treated by removal of the nail and simply allowing it to regrow. If this fails, ablation of the nail bed and avulsion of the nail produces good results (Zadik's operation).

167 A **False** B **True** C **True** D **False** E **True**

Trendelenburg's test is performed by asking the patient to stand on the affected limb. In a positive test, the opposite buttock drops down whereas in the negative test, the buttock rises slightly as the gluteus medius contracts to raise the pelvis and brings the trunk more directly over the limb which is carrying the body weight. The usual causes of a positive test include a congenital dislocation of the hip, poliomyelitis, coxa vara and pain from osteoarthritis and is due to inefficient function of the gluteal muscles.

Questions (*Answers overleaf*)

168 Following a high tibial osteotomy, a patient develops a complete common peroneal nerve palsy. On examination
- **A** sensation over the medial aspect of the calf will be absent
- **B** dorsiflexion of the ankle will be absent
- **C** the patient will still be able to evert the foot
- **D** the great toe extensor will still be active
- **E** plantarflexion of the foot will be weak

169 An arthrogram of the hip would be useful in the diagnosis of
- **A** an intra-articular cartilaginous loose body
- **B** septic arthritis of the hip
- **C** a suspected loose cemented total hip replacement
- **D** a slipped upper femoral epiphysis
- **E** Perthe's disease

170 Spontaneous rupture of the long head of the biceps
- **A** is associated with rheumatoid disease of the shoulder
- **B** most frequently occurs in adolescent males
- **C** produces profound weakness of flexion of the elbow
- **D** should be repaired by a tendon graft in the elderly
- **E** produces the classical physical sign of 'bunching' of the biceps muscle when the elbow is actively flexed

Answers

168 A **False** B **True** C **False** D **False** E **False**

A complete common peroneal nerve palsy is a recognised complication of a high tibial osteotomy. In the majority, the lesion is in continuity and recovers over a period of months. The clinical signs include the inability to dorsiflex the foot due to inactivity of tibialis anterior, the long and short toe extensors. The peronei will be affected resulting in inability to evert the foot. Inversion will take place due to an active tibialis posterior. Sensation in the cleft between the great and second toe will be impaired and also skin over the lateral side of the calf in the lower two-thirds.

169 A **True** B **False** C **True** D **False** E **False**

In arthrography of the hip, radiopaque dye is injected into the joint under sterile conditions, together with a few millilitres of air to produce contrast between the hip architecture and the dye. The technique is useful in children and infants, to outline the articular cartilage and radiolucent areas of the unossified femoral head in congenital dislocation of the hip and Perthe's disease for example, but is not necessary for diagnosis. Cartilaginous loose bodies may be identified by arthrography and also loosening of the components of total hip replacement. In neither septic arthritis or slipped upper femoral epiphysis is an arthrography likely to be a beneficial aid to diagnosis.

170 A **True** B **False** C **False** D **False** E **True**

While spontaneous rupture of the long head of biceps may occur after violent exercise in a young patient, it occurs more frequently in the older age groups. Many are associated with attrition of the tendon by osteophytes around the glenoid or by synovial infiltration in rheumatoid disease. Clinically, there is usually no obvious weakness of elbow flexion, nor does the patient complain of pain. The patient may, however, notice bulging of the biceps on flexing the elbow. In the majority, operative treatment is not required. Occasionally the distal part of the tendon may be sutured to the bicipital groove.

Questions (*Answers overleaf*)

171 Common sites of stress fractures are

- **A** Lower third of tibia
- **B** Midshaft of radius
- **C** Midshaft of fifth metatarsal
- **D** Proximal phalanx of the hand
- **E** The scaphoid

172 Recurrent anterior dislocation of the shoulder

- **A** is invariably associated with a history of acute trauma with each dislocation
- **B** may be associated with a tear between the labrum and the bony glenoid
- **C** is usually caused by external rotation and abduction of the arm
- **D** is most frequent beyond the fourth decade of life
- **E** becomes more painful with increasing frequency of dislocation

173 A fixed equinus of the ankle may be caused by

- **A** cerebral palsy
- **B** spina bifida
- **C** a chronic rupture of the tendo achillis
- **D** Dupuytren's contracture
- **E** congenital metatarsus varus

Answers

171 A **True** B **False** C **False** D **False** E **False**

A stress fracture is one in which a bone is subject to repeated load with excessive frequency resulting in bone failure. Radiographic examination may be normal initially and will later demonstrate periosteal elevation at the site of the fracture. The commonest sites for stress fractures are the second and third metatarsals, described as March fractures and lower third of tibia in joggers. It should be emphasised that any bone undergoing excessive repeated loading may eventually fail.

172 A **False** B **True** C **True** D **False** E **False**

Recurrent anterior dislocation of the shoulder, which occurs in the younger age group, more frequently in males than females, is usually associated with a specific history of acute trauma to the shoulder in the first instance. However, subsequent dislocations may result from trivial injury. A defect antero-inferiorly between the glenoid and the cartilaginous labrum (the Bankart lesion) which fails to heal is one cause of recurrent dislocation, but other sites of weakness include the anterior capsule which is either ruptured or stretched and damage to the subscapularis muscle with overlies the head of the humerus. With increasing frequency of dislocation, pain becomes less of a problem, while instability increases, presumably due to further stretching of damaged structures.

173 A **True** B **True** C **False** D **False** E **False**

A position of fixed plantarflexion of the ankle may occur in several conditions. Neurological conditions in which the ankle plantarflexors are overactive compared to the dorsiflexors include cerebral palsy, spina bifida and hemiplegia from a cerebrovascular accident. Underdevelopment of the calf muscles in congenital talipes equino-varus results in an equinus deformity. Trauma resulting in either fibrosis in the plantarflexor muscles or capsular and bone injury around the ankle may result in a fixed ankle equinus. Although Dupuytren's contracture may occur in the foot, it does not cause an equinus deformity. In congenital metatarsus varus, the deformity occurs in the forefoot and the hindfoot is not affected. Rupture of the tendo achillis results in weakness of plantarflexion.

Questions (*Answers overleaf*)

174 A compression fracture of the vertebral body caused by minor injury may be associated with
- **A** Cushing's disease
- **B** osteoporosis
- **C** a solitary myeloma
- **D** a haemangioma
- **E** osteoarthritis of the lumbar spine

175 Radiological Perthes-like changes in the capital epiphyses of a 9 year old male may be due to
- **A** scurvy
- **B** hyperthyroidism
- **C** multiple epiphyseal dysplasia
- **D** fibrous dysplasia
- **E** Gaucher's disease

176 Polymyalgia rheumatica is associated with
- **A** a normal erythrocyte sedimentation rate
- **B** pain and stiffness around both shoulder and pelvic girdles
- **C** a sensory deficit in specific nerve roots
- **D** sudden blindness
- **E** arthritis of the terminal interphalangeal joints of the fingers

177 Pigmented villo-nodular synovitis
- **A** occurs only in synovial joints
- **B** is more common in females
- **C** contains large amounts of haemosiderin
- **D** is much commoner in haemophiliacs compared to the normal population
- **E** can be excised without fear of local recurrence

Answers

174 A **True** B **True** C **True** D **True** E **False**

Minor injuries to the spine may be the cause of a compression fracture of the vertebrae when there is an underlying bone weakness. This may be caused by osteoporosis which is either idiopathic or due to prolonged steroid therapy and Cushing's syndrome. Tumours, either benign or malignant, which cause bone weakness may result in vertebral collapse. These include secondary deposits, myeloma, and haemangiomata. Metabolic bone disease including osteomalacia may also result in vertebral collapse. Osteoarthritis of the spine is associated with increased bone density and strength.

175 A **False** B **False** C **True** D **False** E **True**

Irregular ossification of the capital epiphysis of the hip may occur in other disorders apart from Perthe's disease. The changes may be seen in multiple epiphyseal dysplasia, usually affecting both hips and other joints including the elbow, knees and ankles. They also occur in cretinism (hypothyroidism), Sickle cell disease, rickettsial infections and Gaucher's disease. A careful history and investigation should allow the clinician to differentiate the causes of the disorder.

176 A **False** B **True** C **False** D **True** E **False**

Polymyalgia rheumatica occurs most commonly in the over 60 year age group and is a self-limiting disease, lasting up to 2 years. It causes severe pain and stiffness of the muscles of the shoulder and pelvic girdles. Joint swelling is not a feature of the disease. The erythrocyte sedimentation rate may be very high, but all other tests are normal. A vasculitis may be found in up to 25% of patients and may cause blindness when affecting the optic artery. Treatment is by high dose steroid therapy.

177 A **False** B **True** C **True** D **False** E **False**

Pigmented villonodular synovitis is seen most frequently in relation to tendon sheaths, joints, occasionally bursae and within cancellous bone near a joint. The disease is approximately three times more common in females. The inflamed synovium contains deposits of haemosiderin probably due to haemorrhage. However, the synovitis does not appear to be commoner in haemophiliacs than the normal population. Despite wide excision of the lesion, local recurrence does occur.

Questions (*Answers overleaf*)

178 The following are positive supportive signs of a recent torn medial meniscus of the knee joint
- **A** An effusion
- **B** An inability to fully extend the knee
- **C** Retropatellar tenderness
- **D** The circumference of the quadriceps muscle increases
- **E** Medial joint line tenderness

179 Congenital syphilis
- **A** is caused by *Treponema pallidum*
- **B** presents with anaemia, wasting, restlessness and fever
- **C** is associated with bilateral painless joint effusions
- **D** results in a diffuse periostitis with periosteal elevation seen on the radiographs
- **E** cannot be treated by antibiotics

180 Avascular necrosis of the upper femoral epiphysis may be caused by
- **A** fracture through the neck of the femur
- **B** slipped upper femoral epiphysis
- **C** septic arthritis of the hip
- **D** fracture of the tibia and fibula
- **E** juvenile diabetes

Answers

178 A **True**
B **True**
C **False**
D **False**
E **True**

While some torn menisci may cause vague symptoms within the knee including recurrent effusions and generalised pain, many result in typical signs which make diagnosis reasonably certain. There may be medial joint line tenderness, an effusion and inability to fully extend the knee. In other words the knee may be locked. Forced full flexion may be painful along the affected joint line or at the back of the knee. McMurray's test may be positive in a torn bucket handle which lies within the intercondylar notch. Because the knee joint fails to function normally, the quadriceps bulk decreases.

179 A **True**
B **True**
C **True**
D **True**
E **False**

An infected mother may transmit the organism *Treponema pallidum,* across the placenta to the fetus. The infected newborn will present with anaemia, fever, wasting and irritability. There may be skin eruptions with moist lesions around the mouth and anus. Long bones around the metaphyseal areas are infiltrated with granulation tissue and a diffuse periostitis may be present resulting in painful swollen limbs. At a later stage, bilateral painless effusions may be seen in the knee joints (Clutton's joints), together with gummatous ulcerations of the skull and long bones. Early treatment with appropriate antibiotics is essential to reduce the long-term effects of the disease.

180 A **True**
B **True**
C **True**
D **False**
E **False**

Avascular necrosis of the upper femoral epiphysis is a serious complication of many hip disorders. They include infections in and around the hip joint, fracture of the neck of the femur, traumatic dislocation of the hip and slipped upper femoral epiphysis. It can also be due to increased pressure on the hip joint caused by manipulation to reduce congenital dislocation of the hip. Perthe's disease of the hip is believed to be due to repeated interruption of the blood supply to the upper end of the femur resulting in areas of avascular necrosis. Rarer causes in children include sickle cell disease and Gaucher's disease.

Questions (*Answers overleaf*)

181 The following muscles are hip extensors
- **A** Obturator internus
- **B** Adductor magnus
- **C** Gluteus medius
- **D** Gluteus maximus
- **E** Biceps femoris

182 A 70 year old male develops symptoms of prostatism, anaemia and bone pain. On rectal examination he has a hard small prostate. Which of the following will help to confirm the diagnosis of carcinoma of the prostate?
- **A** Serum acid phosphatase
- **B** A bone scan
- **C** Plasma proteins
- **D** A skeletal survey
- **E** Prostatic biopsy

183 Acromegaly
- **A** is caused by a tumour or hyperplasia of the posterior pituitary
- **B** results in abnormal thickening of long bones
- **C** appears after skeletal maturity
- **D** may be treated by total body irradiation
- **E** is invariably a rapidly fatal disease

Answers

181 A **False** B **True** C **False** D **True** E **True**

The muscles producing hip extension are the gluteus maximus and the hamstrings (semimembranosus, semitendinosus and biceps femoris). Part of adductor magnus which originates from the ischial tuberosity and inserts into the adductor tubercle also acts as a hip extensor. That part of the muscle together with the hamstrings is supplied by the sciatic nerve, the rest by the obturator. Obturator internus acts as a stabiliser of the hip and a lateral rotator. Gluteus medius acts as an abductor and by its anterior fibres, an internal rotator of the hip joint.

182 A **True** B **True** C **False** D **True** E **True**

Carcinoma of the prostate may be confirmed directly by prostatic biopsy. Since the tumour tends to metastasise early, bone scans and skeletal surveys may show evidence of bone secondaries especially in the pelvic and lumbar regions. Bone secondaries tend to be sclerotic and have a typical appearance on radiographs. In most tumours, the serum acid phosphatase will be raised, though in small tumours and those with a low metabolic activity the level may be normal.

183 A **False** B **True** C **True** D **False** E **False**

Acromegaly is characterised by an unevenly distributed exaggeration of ossification. It is due to production of an excessive amount of growth hormone from the eosinophilic cells of the anterior lobe of the pituitary. Clinically there is increased thickness of the long bones, jaw, ribs and vertebrae. The skull is thickened, especially the frontal bones and the pituitary fossa may be widened. Treatment is directed to the pituitary abnormality of hyperplasia or tumour by surgery or local irradiation. Complications of acromegaly include the carpal tunnel syndrome and degenerative arthritis in the limb and spinal joints.

Questions (*Answers overleaf*)

184 Congenital pseudarthrosis of the tibia
- **A** is associated with neurofibromatosis
- **B** is a common condition
- **C** presents with antero-lateral bowing of the tibia
- **D** is usually bilateral
- **E** can be invariably successfully treated by a cancellous bone graft

185 A high serum calcium may be seen in
- **A** hyperparathyroidism
- **B** malignant bone secondaries
- **C** primary osteoporosis
- **D** vitamin D intoxication
- **E** malabsorption syndromes

186 Acrylic cement, commonly used in total joint replacement
- **A** is a polymer of methylmethacrylate
- **B** results in an endothermic reaction when the liquid is mixed with the powder
- **C** takes about 30 minutes to harden once the liquid is mixed with the powder
- **D** is relatively inert when fixed into the medullary canal of a bone
- **E** is radiopaque

Answers

184 A **True** B **False** C **True** D **False** E **False**

Congenital pseudarthrosis of the tibia is a rare disorder in which a fracture through the tibia fails to heal. It is associated with antero-lateral bowing of the tibia in which there is narrowing of the bone with obliteration of the medullary canal or with a cyst within the bone due to fibrous dysplasia or neurofibromatosis. Bilateral involvement is very rare, in some there is a familial tendency. The tibia alone or more commonly the tibia and fibula may be involved, with the commonest site at the junction between middle and lower thirds. Treatment is difficult and by no means universally successful. Operative procedures include bone grafting, intramedullary nailing and free microvascular fibular grafts. In some children, repeated failure to unite the bone may lead to below-knee amputation.

185 A **True** B **True** C **False** D **True** E **False**

There are many causes of a disturbed calcium metabolism. Hyperparathyroidism resulting in increased renal reabsorption, and bone resorption and intestinal absorption produces a raised serum calcium. Some neoplastic diseases with bone infiltration may cause hypercalcaemia. Vitamin D overdose results in excess intestinal absorption of calcium and thyrotoxicosis may also produce hypercalcaemia by bone resorption.

186 A **True** B **False** C **False** D **True** E **False**

The basis of the use of self-curing acrylic cement is the change from a soft dough-like material to a hard solid material by polymerisation of methylmethacrylate. The dough is made by mixing a liquid containing monomeric methylmethacrylate and an inhibitor, with a powder which contains pre-polymerised methylmethacrylate and an activator which react by an exothermic reaction to produce polymethylmethacrylate. The reaction takes about 7 minutes to occur but may be a little shorter or longer depending on environmental conditions. Fixation of cement and bone depends purely on mechanical interlocking. Additives such as barium to make the cement radiopaque slightly weaken the cement, but providing quantities are small this is not significant. Large pieces of cement are inert in vivo, but very small fragments may produce a granulomatous foreign body reaction which can result in loosening of the cement–bone interface.

Questions (*Answers overleaf*)

187 Kienbock's disease of the wrist
- **A** most frequently occurs in children
- **B** is usually bilateral
- **C** may result in degenerative arthritis of the wrist
- **D** is a disorder without clinical significance
- **E** is caused by an inborn error of metabolism

188 Friedrich's ataxia
- **A** frequently leads to death in the third decade
- **B** usually presents at birth
- **C** is associated with pes planus
- **D** presents with clumsiness of the hands, nystagmus and dysarthria
- **E** does not have a familial tendency

189 Acute anterior poliomyelitis
- **A** frequently presents with a febrile illness
- **B** is caused by a Gram negative bacteria
- **C** affects the anterior horn cells and less frequently the posterior columns of the spinal cord
- **D** has been eradicated from Britain
- **E** affects the lower limbs more frequently than the upper limbs

Answers

187 A **False** B **False** C **True** D **False** E **False**

Fragmentation of the lunate with subsequent degenerative changes in the adjacent joints, is described as Kienbock's disease. Aetiology is not clear. It has been described as one of the osteochondritides, but differs from many others in that it only occurs after maturity. Occasionally the bone may reform but more frequently the fragmentation persists and degenerative changes develop resulting in the symptoms of pain, swelling and instability of the wrist. Treatment of persistent symptoms is by silastic replacement or arthrodesis of the wrist.

188 A **True** B **False** C **False** D **True** E **False**

Friedrich's ataxia is a familial disorder in which inheritance may be recessive or dominant. The disease usually develops between 5 years of age and puberty. The main symptoms are related to cerebellar ataxia producing clumsiness of the hands and subsequently the cortico-spinal tracts become involved. Neurological examination will reveal impaired position and vibration sense, absent tendon reflexes with extensor plantar responses, inco-ordination of the limbs and nystagmus. Many patients develop pes cavus and occasionally a severe scoliosis. In time, cardiomyopathy and dementia may develop and with progress of the disease, frequently leading to death in the third decade.

189 A **True** B **False** C **False** D **False** E **True**

Acute anterior poliomyelitis is an infectious disease caused by the poliovirus which may be ingested in contaminated food and water and primarily becomes established in the intestinal wall and lymph nodes. Via the blood stream, it reaches the anterior horn cells of the spinal cord which may be completely or temporarily damaged resulting in a flaccid paralysis of the affected muscles, with the lower limbs being twice as frequently affected as the upper limbs. Despite immunisation regimes, poliomyelitis still occurs in Britian. It is often in the adult who contracts the disease abroad and has not had a 'booster' dose of live attenuated virus for many years.

Questions (*Answers overleaf*)

190 Recognised complications of a chronic slipped upper femoral epiphysis include
A avascular necrosis of the upper femoral epiphysis
B articular cartilage necrosis
C spontaneous fusion of the hip
D a fixed external rotation deformity of the hip
E a positive Trendelenberg test

191 Regarding swellings at the front of the knee
A the pre-patellar bursa lies between the skin and the patella
B the superficial infrapatella bursa lies between the patella tendon and the skin
C a semimembranosus bursa is the commonest swelling in children
D the pre-patellar bursa communicates with the knee joint in the majority of patients
E the supra-patellar bursa communicates with the knee joint in the vast majority of adults

192 Paraplegia may be caused by the following
A Secondary malignant deposits in the spine
B Spinal artery thrombosis
C Pyogenic extradural abscess
D Fracture-dislocation of the fifth-sixth cervical vertebrae
E Lead poisoning

Answers

190 A **True**
B **True**
C **False**
D **True**
E **True**

Chronic slipped upper femoral epiphysis may be complicated by avascular necrosis spontaneously or due to excessive pressure on the joint when a manual reduction of the slip is attempted. There is now little doubt that a reduction of the slip cannot be performed by manipulation. Necrosis of the articular cartilage is a further complication which may develop spontaneously resulting in a poor prognosis. In a major chronic slip, a fixed external rotation deformity will be apparent as will a positive Trendelenberg test due to weakening of the abductors. Spontaneous fusion of the hip is not a recognised complication of the disorder.

191 A **True**
B **True**
C **False**
D **False**
E **True**

Swellings at the front of the knee are common problems of differential diagnosis. In front of the patella lies the pre-patellar bursa and in front of the patellar ligament lies the superficial infra-patellar bursa. When swollen, the former is called 'Housemaids knee', the latter 'Clergymans knee'. The suprapatellar bursa, which communicates with the knee joint, can result in a large swelling at the front of the knee. A semimembranosus bursa lies within the popliteal fossa. Neither the pre-patellar or infrapatellar bursae communicate with the knee joint.

192 A **True**
B **True**
C **True**
D **False**
E **False**

Surprisingly paraplegia, especially of insidious onset, frequently fails to be diagnosed in the early stages. Either the patient is thought to be malingering or important physical signs are not elicited and obvious ones such as acute retention thought to be due to some other cause such as prostatic hypertrophy. Acute paraplegia most commonly occurs following trauma, rarer causes may be vascular in origin and include anterior spinal thrombosis. Subacute causes include abscesses and secondary carcinoma of the spine. Paraplegia of insidious onset include spinal cord tumours and cervical spondylosis. In children, congenital abnormalities including spina bifida may result in paraplegia. While lead poisoning may cause a peripheral neuropathy, it does not cause paraplegia. A high cervical cord lesion would produce a quadripelgia.

Questions (*Answers overleaf*)

193 Peripheral neuropathy may be caused by
A alcoholism
B vitamin B_{12} deficiency
C diabetes
D excess penicillin ingestion
E lead poisoning

194 Syringomyelia
A most frequently affects the upper limbs
B results in loss of sensation of pain and temperature with retention of light touch and postural sensibility
C results in increased tendon reflexes in the affected limb
D is derived from the Greek words, syrinx, a tube and myelos, the spinal cord
E may be associated with an arthropathy in the upper limbs

195 Which of the following are sesamoid bones?
A The fabella
B The coronoid process
C The pisiform
D The trapezium
E The patella

Answers

193
A **True**
B **True**
C **True**
D **False**
E **True**

In any patient with sensory changes or muscular weakness affecting several peripheral nerves, the differential diagnosis includes peripheral neuropathy. Peripheral neuropathy may be caused by infective disorders such as the Guillain-Barre syndrome and leprosy, metabolic causes including Vitamin B_{12} and Vitamin B_1 deficiency (Beriberi), alcoholism, poisons including heavy metals, lead, arsenic, copper and mercury, diabetes, and rarer causes including carcinomatosis.

194
A **True**
B **True**
C **False**
D **True**
E **True**

Syringomyelia, derived from the Greek 'syrinx' a tube and 'myelos', the spinal cord, is characterised by a cavity within the spinal cord which sometimes passes up to the medulla resulting in syringobulbia. In syringomyelia, there is slow onset of wasting of muscles of the hand, together with loss of sensation of pain and temperature. Appreciation of light touch and postural sensibility are preserved (dissociated sensory loss). It occurs because the central syrinx damages the fibres which decussate while the fibres in the posterior columns are unaffected. The anterior horn cells are directly compressed resulting in a lower motor lesion with diminished or absent reflexes. A neuropathic arthropathy may develop in the shoulders and elbows of some patients with syringomyelia.

195
A **True**
B **False**
C **True**
D **False**
E **True**

Sesamoid bones are more or less rounded nodules of bone imbedded in certain tendons and are usually related to articular surfaces. They probably act to modify direction of muscle pull, the patella for example, or to diminish friction or to modify pressure. The hand has several sesamoid bones including one in the tendon of adductor pollicis and one in flexor pollicis brevis. The pisiform fulfills the criteria of a sesamoid bone but is described as a carpal bone. The patella is the largest sesamoid bone in the body. The fabella, within the lateral head of gastrocnemius is important in that it may be mistaken for a loose body within the knee joint.

Questions (*Answers overleaf*)

196 Concerning the bony articulations in the foot
- **A** The talus articulates with the cuboid bone
- **B** The cuneiform bones, two in number, articulate with the anterior border of the navicular bone
- **C** The calcaneum articulates with the talus at the subtalar joint
- **D** Each cuneiform bone has a metatarsal articulating with its anterior border
- **E** The lateral cuneiform articulates with the cuboid

197 Cervical spondylosis
- **A** most frequently affects the upper vertebrae
- **B** produces pain and paraesthesiae over the lateral aspect of the forearm and thumb when affecting the sixth cervical nerve
- **C** may produce an upper motor neurone lesion in the lower limbs
- **D** most frequently results from an incident of acute trauma
- **E** may cause occipital headaches

Answers

196 A **False** B **False** C **True** D **True** E **True**

The calcaneum articulates with the talus at the subtalar joint. The cuboid articulates with the anterior part of the calcaneum and the navicular with the head of the talus anteriorly. The three cuneiforms fill the gap on the medial side of the foot in front of the navicular and the medial side of the anterior part of the cuboid. Two metatarsals articulate with the front of the cuboid and the medial three metatarsals with each of the three cuneiforms.

197 A **False** B **True** C **True** D **False** E **True**

Cervical spondylosis is a syndrome in which pain in the cervical region, associated with pain and paraesthesiae in the upper limbs is due to intervertebral disc degeneration and facet joint arthritis. The degenerative changes result in pain from the joint degeneration and also from nerve impingement at the foramina. The site of paraesthesia and neurological signs depends on which nerve roots are involved. For example, irritation of the second cervical nerve will produce occipital pain while the sixth cervical nerve irritation produces symptoms in the forearm and thumb. The lower vertebrae are more frequently involved than the upper. In the upper limbs, muscle weakness is due to a lower motor neurone disorder since the peripheral nerves are involved. In the lower limbs, an upper motor lesion may be present since osteophyte formation damages the cord itself. Most patients develop the pathological changes spontaneously, though localised changes may be secondary to trauma.

Questions (*Answers overleaf*)

198 Complications of prolonged steroid therapy for rheumatoid arthritis include
A osteoporosis
B depression of ACTH pituitary secretion
C pathological fractures
D a rise in serum potassium
E cutaneous striae and moon facies

199 Volkmann's ischaemic contracture
A results in fixed contractures of the flexor muscles of the forearm
B is solely the effect of ischaemia on the median and ulnar nerves
C may be precipitated by a displaced supracondylar fracture of the elbow
D is a type of compartment syndrome
E results in hyperextension of the wrist and clawing of the fingers

200 Increased bone density in a vertebral body on radiographic examination may be due to
A a haemangioma
B crush fracture
C myeloma
D prostatic secondaries
E Paget's disease

Answers

198 A **True** B **True** C **True** D **False** E **True**

Corticosteroids are used to suppress the inflammatory component of the synovitis in rheumatoid arthritis. Systemic complications are many including depression of pituitary ACTH secretion and atrophy of the adrenal cortices. The patient develops Cushingoid features including a moon face, cutaneous striae and increased deposition of subcutaneous fat especially round the shoulders. Bone becomes osteoporotic due partly to the catabolic affect of steroids and pathological fractures may occur. There may be electrolytic disturbances with a fall in the serum potassium causing cardiac arrhythmias. The serum sodium rises in the early stages with water retention. Steroids are diabetogenic and result in an increase in insulin requirements in diabetics.

199 A **True** B **False** C **True** D **True** E **False**

Volkmann's ischaemic contracture, originally described in 1881, is characterised by ischaemic necrosis of the structures within the volar aspect of the forearm. Muscle necrosis results in contracture from fibrosis with subsequent flexion contracture of the wrist and fingers. The ulnar and median nerves may be damaged either by direct ischaemia or compression by adjacent fibrous tissue. The syndrome is caused by ischaemia, usually following trauma to the region of the elbow. Circulation to the forearm is decreased or completely severed. The muscles within the tight fascial compartments of the forearm swell, further decreasing circulation and a vicious circle of muscle swelling and circulatory impairment is set in motion. This disorder is termed a compartment syndrome.

200 A **False** B **True** C **False** D **True** E **True**

Increased bone density in a vertebral body is an uncommon, though recurrent problem of diagnosis. It may be caused by several unrelated conditions. Pagets disease with a cotton wool-like condensation of the body, also results in enlargement of the vertebral body. Metastases from the prostate produce increased bone density. In children, Calves disease (vertebra plana) causes increased density of the vertebral body which also become flattened. A crush fracture appears denser than surrounding bone due to the condensation of the trabeculae. A haemangioma of the vertebral body results in a honeycomb appearance or cranio-caudal striations.

Trauma

Questions (*Answers overleaf*)

201 The early clinical signs and symptoms of ischaemia in the forearm and hand following closed reduction of a supracondylar fracture in children are

A Paralysis of the median nerve
B Gangrene of the tips of the fingers
C Fixed contracture of the flexor muscles
D Pain, especially on extension of the fingers
E Absent radial pulse and poor capillary return

202 In an acute rupture of the tendo-achillis in a 40 year old sports man

A there is often a history of direct injury to the heel
B compression of the calf muscle results in plantar flexion of the foot
C diagnosis can be made on radiological examination
D treatment may be conservative using an above-knee plaster, with the ankle dorsiflexed
E operative repair of the rupture may be perfomed with application of an above knee plaster with the ankle plantarflexed

203 The following are complications of a Colles fracture of the wrist

A Rupture of the extensor tendon of the thumb
B Frequent non-union of the fracture
C Median nerve compression
D Mal-union
E Inferior radio-ulnar subluxation

Answers

201 A **False** B **False** C **False** D **True** E **True**

The early symptoms of ischaemia in the forearm following reduction are continued pain on removing all restricting dressings including a plaster, or pain on passive extension of the fingers. Occasionally an absent radial pulse may be found with a good capillary circulation, but an absent pulse with poor capillary return are signs of circulatory obstruction. Paralysis from nerve ischaemia, gangrene of the finger tips and contractures of the flexor muscles are all late signs of ischaemia and are all irreversible.

202 A **False** B **False** C **False** D **False** E **True**

In acute rupture of the tendo-achillis, the patient may feel that he has been kicked on the heel, but direct injury is rare. Failure of the patient to stand on tiptoe on the affected side and lack of plantarflexion of the foot when the calf muscle is compressed are strong diagnostic signs. Radiographs will provide little information, since the tendo-achillis is radiolucent. Treatment of the acute injury is controversial; some surgeons believe that conservative treatment in an above knee plaster with the ankle plantarflexed for 6–8 weeks produces as good a result as operative repair of the tendon and application of plaster with the ankle plantarflexed.

203 A **True** B **False** C **True** D **True** E **True**

Colles fractures are common injuries, yet serious complications are infrequent. The commonest incidence is mal-union, sometimes associated with inferior radio-ulnar subluxation and a prominent and painful distal end of ulna. Non-union is very rare. Stiffness of fingers, wrist, elbow and shoulder occur and occasionally Sudek's atrophy in which the bones of the wrist and hand become porotic, the skin swollen and the joints stiff and painful. Spontaneous rupture of the extensor pollicis longus may occur at about 6 weeks from injury and signs and symptoms of median nerve compression are a further documented complication.

Questions (*Answers overleaf*)

204 In a mallet finger injury
- **A** the extensor tendon to the finger may be avulsed along with a fragment of bone from the base of the terminal phalanx
- **B** there may be a pure rupture of the extensor tendon at its insertion into the distal phalanx
- **C** a persistant flexion deformity invariably requires fusion of the distal interphalangeal joint
- **D** the joint should be immobilised in a splint with the terminal interphalangeal joint extended for about 6 weeks
- **E** no treatment apart from a bandage is required

205 An acute anterior dislocation of the shoulder is associated with which of the following complications?
- **A** Axillary nerve injury
- **B** Fracture of the neck of the humerus
- **C** Fracture of the greater tuberosity
- **D** Frequent rupture of the axillary artery
- **E** A compression fracture in the head of the humerus

206 Fatigue or stress fractures are commonly associated with which of the following bones?
- **A** Humerus
- **B** Thumb metacarpal
- **C** Tibia
- **D** 2nd metatarsal
- **E** Fibula

Answers

204 A **True** B **True** C **False** D **True** E **False**

A mallet finger injury is one in which the extensor tendon is torn away from its insertion into the distal phalanx or occasionally a fragment of bone is avulsed with the tendon. Active treatment is necessary to attempt to allow the tendon or fragment of bone to heal without lengthening. Failure of this to occur results in a flexion deformity of approximately 20° or more. With such a result, most patients accept the deformity, but occasionally the inconvenience results in a request for further treatment which may be either an attempt to shorten the tendon or to perform a fusion of the terminal interphalangeal joint.

205 A **True** B **True** C **True** D **False** E **True**

Damage to the axillary nerve, with inability to contract the deltoid muscle and anaesthesia of the skin overlying the muscle (C.5) is a recognised complication of an acute anterior dislocation and must be identified before reduction. A fracture of the greater tuberosity is the commonest associated fracture which may require operative reduction especially in the younger age group since part of the rotator cuff muscles is attached to it. Fracture of the neck of the humerus is a further recognised complication, but rupture of the axillary artery is very rare. A compression fracture of the head of the humerus (the Hill-Sachs lesion) caused by the head hitting the front of the glenoid as it dislocates is well recognised and may be seen on an antero-posterior radiograph with the humerus fully internally rotated.

206 A **False** B **False** C **True** D **True** E **True**

Fatigue fractures are commonly associated with the tibia, the lateral malleolus and the second metatarsal (march fracture). The fracture is associated with repetitive activity rather than a specific injury, resulting in a 'hairline' fracture which presents clinically with pain and swelling though minimal change on initial radiographs. Subsequent radiographs will show callus formation around 3–4 weeks from injury.

Questions (*Answers overleaf*)

207 The following statements associated with recurrent dislocation of the patella are correct

A The disorder is commoner in adolescent boys than girls
B The initial dislocation is often associated with a severe blow to the knee
C The patella usually dislocates medially
D Operative treatment should be performed the first time a patella dislocates to prevent recurrence
E Radiographs are necessary in management of the patient

208 The following fractures usually require open reduction and internal fixation

A An oblique fracture of the midshaft of humerus
B An oblique fracture of the proximal third of the ulna with anterior dislocation of the radial head in an adult
C A pathological fracture of the midshaft of the femur in a 40 year old female with breast carcinoma
D A two-part intertrochanteric fracture in an elderly female
E A displaced fracture of the lateral condyle of the elbow in a 10 year old

209 In a fracture of the calcaneum

A a common immediate clinical sign is an ecchymosis on the plantar surface of the foot
B prognosis is worse when the fracture involves the sub-talar joint, rather than the body of the calcaneum
C the patient may complain of thoracic or lumbar pain
D ankle movements are not usually impaired
E the mid-tarsal joint is never affected by the injury

Answers

207 A **False** B **False** C **False** D **False** E **True**

Recurrent dislocation of the patella is commoner in females than males. The initial dislocation is often associated with a minor injury. The patella almost always dislocates laterally. Most authorities would agree that reduction of the dislocation and rest in a backslab with the knee extended for a period of 4–6 weeks to allow the soft tissues to heal, is preferable to operative treatment initially. Radiographs should be performed to exclude osteochondral fractures produced by shearing of the lateral femoral condyle by the patella and also to identify bony abnormalities within the knee joint.

208 A **False** B **True** C **True** D **True** E **True**

Management of many fractures depends on the attitude of the individual surgeon, but most would agree that the following require open reduction and internal fixation; an oblique fracture of the ulna and dislocation of the radial head, since conservative management may result in loss of position; pathological fractures of long bones, sometimes with the use of bone cement, to relieve pain and allow early mobility; hip fractures in elderly females, to allow early mobilisation and prevent general complications; displaced intra-articular fractures, to allow perfect reduction and decrease the risk of post-traumatic osteoarthritis.

209 A **False** B **True** C **True** D **True** E **False**

Immediate examination following a calcaneal fracture will show swelling and tenderness around the heel. Ankle joint movement will be maintained, but subtalar and midtarsal movements will be restricted and painful. An ecchymosis in the sole of the foot will develop a few days after injury. Since many calcaneal injuries are due to a fall from a height, the patient may also sustain compression injuries of the spine and these must be excluded. Serious calcaneal injuries are those which extend into the sub-talar and mid-tarsal joints, since in many cases, residual stiffness and post-traumatic osteoarthritis will develop.

Questions (*Answers overleaf*)

210 Common complications of inter-trochanteric fractures despite treatment are
- **A** Mal-union
- **B** Non-union
- **C** Coxa vara
- **D** Avascular necrosis of the femoral head
- **E** Sciatic nerve palsy

211 A complete radial nerve palsy associated with a closed fracture of the humerus
- **A** results in an inability to extend the interphalangeal joints of the hand
- **B** results in an inability to extend the wrist
- **C** is most commonly associated with a lesion in continuity
- **D** produces anaesthesia over the dorsum of the hand including the skin over the proximal phalanges of middle and index fingers and thumb
- **E** if showing no sign of recovery at 6 months can be usefully treated by tendon transfer

Answers

210 A **True** Inter-trochanteric fractures rarely result in non-
B **False** union after treatment since the bone involved is
C **True** mainly cancellous and has a good blood supply.
D **False** Mal-union is common following treatment by
E **False** internal fixation or skeletal traction and usually results in coxa vara with subsequent shortening of the affected limb. Sciatic nerve palsy is a very rare complication. Avascular necrosis of the femoral head is rarely associated with an inter-trochanteric fracture since it is extracapsular and does not involve the retinacular vessels.

211 A **False** A complete or partial nerve palsy is a recognised
B **True** complication of midshaft fractures of the humerus
C **True** and is associated with the close relationship
D **False** between bone and nerve in the spiral groove. The
E **True** injury results in an inability to extend the wrist and metacarpo-phalangeal joints, but the interphalangeal joints can be extended by the action of the intrinsic muscles of the hand innervated by the intact ulnar and median nerves. Sensory deficit is often surprisingly little, being characteristically a small area over the dorsal web between thumb and index finger, presumably due to sensory overlap by the other nerves of the hand. Most lesions are in continuity, but if recovery is not apparent by about 6 months, tendon transfers to wrist and finger extensors provide useful function in the hand.

Questions (*Answers overleaf*)

212 In an ulnar nerve paralysis caused by injury at the midhumeral level, you would usually find

A clawing of the two fingers on the ulnar side of the hand
B unimpaired flexion when making a fist
C an impaired ability to pinch with thumb and index finger
D a lack of thumb sensation
E paralysis of the abductor pollicis brevis

213 Fractures of the ribs may be associated with which of the following complications?

A Haemothorax
B Pneumothorax
C Paradoxical breathing
D Surgical emphysema
E Tension pneumothorax

Answers

212 A **True** B **False** C **True** D **False** E **False**

Paralysis of the ulnar nerve at the midhumeral level would result in clawing of the little and ring fingers due to loss of the intrinsic muscles with resultant failure to extend the interphalangeal joints and flex the metacarpo-phalangeal joints. The flexor profundus to the little and ring fingers would be paralysed, thereby reducing the degree of clawing compared to an ulnar nerve lesion distal to the innervation of the flexor profundus. This is called the ulnar paradox since the more proximal lesion appears to produce a less serious deformity. Wrist flexion will be impaired since flexor carpi ulnaris would be paralysed. Pinch grip would be impaired since it requires the first dorsal interosseous muscle and adductor pollicis (ulnar nerve) together with the long thumb flexor (median nerve). Thumb sensation is supplied by the median and radial nerves, the abductor pollicis brevis by the median nerve.

213 A **True** B **True** C **True** D **True** E **True**

Fractures of the ribs are usually caused by direct injury, occasionally by a heavy bout of coughing or sneezing. If displacement of the fragments is marked then the pleura or lung may be pierced resulting in a pneumothorax or haemopneumothorax. Paradoxical breathing may occur following multiple rib fractures resulting in a flail segment of the chest wall. As the patient inspires, the flail segment will collapse due to the negative intra-thoracic pressure while the rest of the chest will expand. Surgical emphysema may occur following rib fracture when injury to the lung results in leakage of air into the subcutaneous tissues. A tension pneumothorax may develop if the pleura is penetrated, since by a valve-like mechanism air enters the pleural cavity on inspiration, but is not released on expiration. An increasing volume of air fills the pleural cavity, pushing the mediastinum across to the opposite side of the chest.

Questions (*Answers overleaf*)

214 A fracture of the carpal scaphoid

- **A** is frequently caused by a fall on the outstretched hand
- **B** usually occurs through the waist of the scaphoid
- **C** may be complicated by avascular necrosis of the distal fragment
- **D** is more commonly found in younger patients than the old
- **E** may be complicated by non-union

215 A Monteggia fracture-dislocation of the forearm

- **A** is a combination of a fracture of the proximal ulna with dislocation of the radial head
- **B** is a combination of a fracture of the radius with dislocation of the distal radio-ulnar joint
- **C** is not seen in children
- **D** can usually be treated conservatively in adults
- **E** is frequently associated with a posterior interosseous nerve palsy

216 Fractures of the clavicle

- **A** usually result from direct injury to the bone
- **B** frequently result in fibrous union which is asymptomatic
- **C** are commonest in the middle third of the bone
- **D** in adults, usually require open reduction and internal fixation when the fracture is displaced
- **E** can usually be treated symptomatically by a broad arm sling in children

Answers

214 A **True** B **True** C **False** D **True** E **True**

Carpal scaphoid fractures commonly occur in young adults. They are usually caused by a fall onto the outstretched hand or 'kick-back' when using a starting handle on a motor engine. Over 90% of scaphoid fractures occur through the waist or in the proximal part of the scaphoid. The blood supply to the scaphoid is through multiple small foramina in the distal part of the bone. With a fracture through the waist or proximal pole, the blood supply may be cut off from the proximal part resulting in avascular necrosis. Non-union of a fracture of the scaphoid is a well recognised complication.

215 A **True** B **False** C **False** D **False** E **False**

A Monteggia fracture-dislocation of the forearm comprises of a fracture of the upper end of the ulna with dislocation of the head of the radius. An anterior dislocation is more common than a posterior dislocation. It may occur in children with an apparently minimally displaced greenstick fracture of the ulna due to the elasticity of the bone which at the time of injury may bend markedly only to return to its original shape. The radial head, remains dislocated. A line drawn along the shaft of the radius should pass through the capitellum when the head is normally located. Accurate reduction is essential with maintenance of position of the fracture to ensure reduction of the radial head within the annular ligament. In adults, internal fixation of the ulna is strongly advised. Surprisingly, injury to the posterior interosseous nerve as it passes around the neck of the radius, is not a common complication.

216 A **False** B **False** C **True** D **False** E **True**

Fractures of the clavicle are usually caused by a fall on the outstretched hand. They occur most commonly at the middle third of the bone. Non-union of the fracture is rare. Treatment in both adults and children is aimed at relieving pain by resting the shoulder using a broad arm sling and reducing the fracture by bracing the shoulders backward using a figure-of-eight bandage. In children, simply using a broad arm sling to relieve pressure on the clavicle is often sufficient treatment.

Questions (*Answers overleaf*)

217 Recognised complications of closed midshaft fractures of the humerus include
- **A** non-union
- **B** axillary nerve palsy
- **C** radial nerve palsy
- **D** musculo-cutaneous nerve palsy
- **E** frequent rupture of the brachial artery

218 In fractures of the odontoid process of the axis
- **A** sudden death is the usual outcome
- **B** the odontoid usually lies anterior to the body of the axis
- **C** the injury is most easily seen on the routine antero-posterior radiograph
- **D** displaced fractures should be treated initially by skull traction under radiographic control
- **E** a late presentation of a displaced odontoid fracture may be increasing long tract signs

219 Complications of pelvic fractures include
- **A** haemorrhage
- **B** rupture of the bladder
- **C** rupture of the urethra
- **D** osteoarthritis of the hip
- **E** leg length discrepancy

Answers

217 A **True**
B **False**
C **True**
D **False**
E **False**

Closed midshaft fractures of the humerus are associated with radial nerve lesions, since the nerve is bound onto the spiral groove by the triceps muscle. The midshaft of the humerus is a well recognised site for delayed and non-union although the complication is uncommon. Rupture of the brachial artery is a very rare complication of a midshaft fracture.

218 A **False**
B **True**
C **False**
D **True**
E **True**

A fracture of the odontoid may be caused by a flexion injury to the neck with forward displacement of the odontoid or more rarely by an extension injury in which the odontoid is displaced posteriorly. While sudden death may occur from the injury due to cord damage, the numbers of patients presenting in casualty suggest that this is not the usual outcome. The patient is seen to support his head in his hands and may complain that his 'head feels that it is falling off'. Diagnosis depends on radiological examination and will show up best on the transoral and lateral cervical view. Lateral flexion-extension views under careful supervision may be necessary. Initial treatment is usually by skull traction to reduce the displacement, followed by a plaster jacket with head support or well fitting collar. Non-union of the odontoid fracture or delayed diagnosis may result in the patient presenting with late signs of cord compression.

219 A **True**
B **True**
C **True**
D **True**
E **True**

Complications following pelvic fractures may include severe haemorrhage both from soft tissue damage and rupture of main vessels by bone fragments. Rupture of the bladder, by indirect pressure of the injury on a full bladder or by direct bony injury is well recognised. Urethral damage is associated with double fractures of the ischial and pubic rami or by disruption of the symphysis pubis. Inability to pass urine and blood at the urethral meatus demands further radiological and urological investigation. Pelvic fractures into the acetabulum may lead to secondary osteoarthritis of the hip joint. Marked upward displacement of one hemipelvis, caused by a fracture through both the anterior and posterior aspects of the pelvic ring, will lead to a leg length discrepancy if not reduced.

Questions (*Answers overleaf*)

220 In a posterior dislocation of the hip
- **A** the affected limb is flexed, externally rotated and adducted
- **B** the affected limb is flexed, internally rotated and adducted
- **C** there may be an associated fracture of the femoral head
- **D** recurrent dislocation is a frequent complication despite satisfactory treatment
- **E** the injury may result from the flexed knee impacting against the dashboard of the car in a road traffic accident

221 Complications of a posterior dislocation of the hip include
- **A** avascular necrosis of the head of the femur
- **B** myositis ossificans
- **C** sciatic nerve palsy
- **D** lateral popliteal nerve palsy
- **E** fracture of the neck of the femur

222 Concerning fractures in the foot
- **A** A fracture at the base of the 5th metatarsal is frequently an avulsion injury
- **B** Displaced fractures of the neck of the talus may be complicated by avascular necrosis
- **C** Most displaced talar neck fractures can be reduced by dorsiflexing the forefoot
- **D** A stress fracture of the 2nd metatarsal may not be obvious on initial radiographic examination
- **E** Fractures of the metatarsals usually require open reduction and internal fixation despite minimal displacement of the fragments

Answers

220 A **False** B **True** C **True** D **False** E **True**

A posterior dislocation of the hip, which may be caused by an impact of the knee against the dashboard of a car with the hip flexed and adducted, presents with an internally rotated, adducted and flexed limb. It is shorter than the opposite normal limb. Following treatment, recurrent dislocation is uncommon. It may occur if a large posterior fragment of the acetabulum is not recognised and treated by open reduction and screw fixation. A fracture of the femoral head is a recognised complication of a posterior dislocation of the hip, although it is uncommon.

221 A **True** B **True** C **True** D **False** E **True**

Avascular necrosis of the head of the femur may complicate dislocation of the hip, due to disruption of the retinacular vessels. Myositis ossificans associated with stiffness of the hip may occur especially after open reduction. Approximately 10% of dislocations are associated with sciatic nerve palsy. The lesion is usually in continuity and will resolve in many cases. Fracture of the neck of the femur may occur, due to initial impact or too forceful reduction of the dislocation.

222 A **True** B **True** C **False** D **True** E **False**

Fractures at the base of the 5th metatarsal are frequently avulsion fractures produced by a sudden pull of the peroneus brevis which is attached at that site. Fractures through the neck of the talus are at risk of avascular necrosis of the body by damage to the nutrient vessels at the time of injury. Plantarflexion of the forefoot will usually reduce moderately displaced fractures. Compression screw fixation has been advocated to reduce the problem of avascular necrosis. Stress fractures in the foot most commonly occur in the 2nd metatarsal. Following prolonged weight bearing (e.g. marching) the patient complains of pain perhaps with localised swelling. Immediate radiographs may be normal, but a subsequent view 2–3 weeks following injury will show callus formation. The majority of metatarsal fractures can be treated conservatively with a below-knee plaster. Only with multiple displaced fractures should open reduction and Kirschner wire fixation be considered.

Questions (*Answers overleaf*)

223 Gamekeeper's thumb

A is rarely seen with the demise of the gamekeeper
B can invariably be diagnosed on routine radiographs
C may be confirmed by stress radiographs of the metacarpophalangeal joint
D is due to rupture of the ulnar collateral ligament of the metacarpophalangeal joint
E results in weakness of pinch grip if not treated

224 The following complications may arise following fracture of the neck of the femur in a 65 year old female

a Non-union in about a quarter of all cases despite competent primary treatment
B Union of the fracture with subsequent avascular necrosis of the head of the femur
C Late osteoarthritis despite union of the fracture
D Failure of diagnosis due to the fact that the patient can straight leg raise in cases of an impacted fracture
E Loss of leg length greater than 10 cm due to mal-union

Answers

223 A **False** B **False** C **True** D **True** E **True**

Rupture of the ulnar collateral ligament of the thumb (Gamekeeper's thumb) is usually caused by forcible abduction of the proximal phalanx against the metacarpal. The eponym is derived from the fact that gamekeepers sustained the injury when wringing the necks of rabbits. A high index of suspicion is necessary for diagnosis which is based on swelling and tenderness over the joint associated with instability of the joint. Routine radiographs are usually normal but occasionally may show a flake of bone pulled off the origin of the ulnar collateral ligament. Stress views may be helpful in confirming diagnosis. If not diagnosed, the patient will complain of a poor pinch grip and pain over the joint. Treatment is either immobilisation in a scaphoid-type plaster for 6 weeks for a partial tear or operative repair for complete tears.

224 A **True** B **True** C **True** D **True** E **False**

Fracture of the neck of the femur is a common injury in the elderly. The diagnosis is usually clear, but occasionally impacted fractures may be missed because the physical signs are minimal. Despite competent primary treatment by internal fixation, about a quarter of all femoral neck fractures fail to unite. Some develop avascular necrosis due to damage of the retinacular vessels as they pass along the neck of the femur. It should be noted that avascular necrosis may occur despite union of the fracture since the blood supply to the head may not be sufficient to stop irreversible changes in the femoral head. Late osteoarthritis, related to damage to the articular cartilage at the time of injury, mal-union or avascular necrosis is a well recognised problem.

Questions (*Answers overleaf*)

225 In fractures of the patella

A inability to extend the knee following a transverse fracture suggests rupture of the quadriceps expansion, providing pain is not severe

B a direct injury to the patella does not usually result in rupture of the quadriceps expansion

C a palpable gap between the upper and lower poles of the patella suggests that the quadriceps expansion has been ruptured

D operative treatment is seldom indicated in displaced transverse fractures

E patellectomy should be performed even in undisplaced fractures to avoid subsequent arthritis

226 In ankle fractures

A external rotation and abduction of the talus relative to the tibia is the commonest mechanism of injury

B isolated fractures of the lateral malleolus or medial malleolus may be treated by plaster immobilisation if undisplaced

C failure to accurately reduce an ankle fracture is an indication for open reduction and internal fixation

D strain-view radiographs may be necessary to demonstrate the extent of ligamentous injury

E osteoarthritis rarely occurs following ankle fractures despite poor reduction

Answers

225 A **True** B **True** C **True** D **False** E **False**

The two essential features in treatment of patella fractures are that the extensor mechanism of the knee must be restored and the articular surface of the patella must be perfectly reconstituted. A direct injury to the patella results in either an undisplaced crack fracture or a comminuted fracture while a displaced transverse fracture is usually caused by an avulsion when the quadriceps are contracted on a flexed knee. Providing the patient can actively extend the knee, the undisplaced fracture can be treated conservatively. A displaced fracture requires open reduction and fixation together with repair of the quadriceps expansion. Patellectomy should only be performed when the articular surface cannot accurately be reduced and where there is a high risk of post-traumatic osteoarthritis.

226 A **True** B **True** C **True** D **True** E **False**

The commonest mechanism of injury in ankle fractures is external rotation and abduction of the talus. Other mechanisms include adduction or vertical compression forces. The true extent of an ankle injury may require strain views under anaesthetic reproducing the mechanism of injury, since following injury the ankle mortice may return to a position that appears normal on routine radiographs and masks features requiring operative treatment. Treatment of ankle fractures is aimed at restoring an anatomical alignment of the articular surfaces and holding the position until bony union or ligament healing occurs. Failure to do so often results in post-traumatic osteoarthritis. Undisplaced fractures may be treated conservatively, but displaced fractures should be treated by open reduction and screw fixation.

Questions (*Answers overleaf*)

227 Concerning fractures in the hand

A A Bennett's fracture is a fracture of the base of the thumb metacarpal not involving the joint
B Isolated undisplaced fractures of the metacarpals seldom need internal fixation
C Displaced intra-articular fractures of the phalanges should be treated by early mobilisation, disregarding the X-ray appearances
D Prolonged immobilisation of the interphalangeal joints in flexion may result in permanent stiffness
E Non-union is a common complication of metacarpal fractures

228 In an anterior cruciate ligament tear of the knee

A the patient may have sustained a hyperextension injury of the knee joint
B Lachman's test will be positive
C there may be an associated tear of the medial meniscus
D the patient will usually have a serious knee disability unless the ligament tear is treated surgically
E a course of intensive isometric quadriceps exercises will relieve symptoms in many patients with a tear of the anterior cruciate

Answers

227 A **False** B **True** C **False** D **True** E **False**

A Bennett's fracture-dislocation occurs at the trapezio-metacarpal joint with the fracture line at the base of the thumb metacarpal entering the joint. While the smaller fragment maintains its alignment with the trapezium, the major fragment subluxates proximally and laterally. Most isolated metacarpal fractures are stable due to splinting by adjacent metacarpals and are treated conservatively. Displaced intra-articular fractures of the phalanges require internal fixation usually by open reduction to reconstitute the articular surface followed by early mobilisation. Prolonged immobilisation of the hand frequently results in joint stiffness. Joints should be mobilised earlier than 3 weeks from injury if possible and if the interphalangeal joints are to be immobilized, it should be in extension to avoid permanent stiffness. Non-union is uncommon in metacarpal fractures despite minimal external splintage.

228 A **True** B **True** C **True** D **False** E **True**

Anterior cruciate tears usually occur from hyperextension of the knee or by a twisting injury as part of the complex of torn medial ligament, anterior cruciate and medial meniscus (O'Donohue's triad). A positive Lachman's test, in which the tibia moves on the femoral condyles in an anterior-posterior plane with the knee flexed approximately 10 to 20 degrees, will be obtained when the anterior cruciate is ruptured. An isolated anterior cruciate tear does not always cause instability severe enough to warrant reconstruction, especially if the quadriceps muscle is fully developed.

Questions (*Answers overleaf*)

229 A Barton's fracture of the wrist is

A a fracture at the distal inch of the radius with palmar displacement of the distal fragment

B a fracture through the distal radius involving the joint and resulting in palmar subluxation of the carpus on the radius

C usually treated conservatively by reduction and application of a Colles-type plaster, since reduction results in stability of the fracture

D usually treated by open reduction and internal fixation in younger patients

E best seen on the lateral radiograph

230 A patient sustains an anterior dislocation of the shoulder joint together with a complete musculocutaneous nerve palsy. Which of the following will be present?

A Diminished sensation of the skin over the deltoid muscle

B Absence of contraction of the biceps muscle

C Decreased power of supination in the forearm

D Decreased sensation over the medial border of the forearm

E Weakness of flexion at the elbow

231 In dislocations of the acromio-clavicular joint

A routine radiographs may not show the full extent of the injury

B complete displacement of the clavicle from the acromion suggests rupture of the conoid and trapezoid ligaments

C the injury is usually caused by a fall onto the outstretched hand

D conservative treatment usually holds the dislocation in a reduced position

E operative repair includes reduction and fixation of the joint together with repair of the disrupted deltoid and trapezius muscle insertions around the joint

Answers

229 A **False** B **True** C **False** D **True** E **True**

A Barton's fracture is a marginal fracture of the palmar surface of the distal end of the radius with radiocarpal subluxation. A fracture at the distal inch of the radius with palmar displacement of the distal fragment is termed a Smith's fracture. Barton's fractures are difficult to hold until union occurs. The optimal position of the wrist to maintain reduction is full supination, with slight dorsiflexion of the wrist and application of an above-elbow plaster. In younger patients accurate reduction is essential both for function and to reduce the risk of osteoarthritis at the wrist. Internal fixation of the fracture is therefore indicated with a buttress plate applied to the palmar surface of the radius.

230 A **False** B **True** C **True** D **False** E **True**

Although palsy of the axillary nerve is the commonest nerve lesion following an anterior dislocation of the shoulder, injury to the musculocutaneous nerve is another recognised complication. The musculocutaneous nerve, which is a branch of the lateral cord of the brachial plexus passes in front of the shoulder joint, through coracobrachialis, between biceps and brachialis supplying all three muscles. On the lateral side of biceps and brachialis in their distal third it emerges as the lateral cutaneous nerve of the forearm to supply the skin as far distally as the ball of the thumb. The patient will have a decreased power of supination since biceps is a powerful supinator.

231 A **True** B **True** C **False** D **False** E **True**

Dislocations of the acromio-clavicular joint are usually caused by a fall onto the outer aspect of the shoulder. Routine radiography of the joint may not reveal the full extent of the injury since following the dislocation the acromion and clavicle may spring back into their normal alignment. An antero-posterior view of both shoulders with the patient holding weights is advisable in suspected cases. A complete displacement of the joint is associated with disruption of the coraco-clavicular ligaments and also part of the insertion of the deltoid and trapezius muscles where they insert into bone around the joint. Conservative treatment often results in failure to hold the joint reduced and operative treatment is advised in most patients.

Questions (*Answers overleaf*)

232 In fractures through the neck of the humerus

A avascular necrosis of the head of the humerus is common
B the fracture may be complicated by an axillary nerve palsy
C open reduction and internal fixation of an undisplaced fracture is necessary because of the high incidence of non-union following conservative treatment
D damage to the brachial plexus may occur in severly displaced fractures
E a single antero-posterior radiograph will provide satisfactory information concerning displacement of the fracture

233 Concerning acute rupture of the tendo achillis

A It is commoner in adolescents than adults
B May be preceded by steroid injections around the tendon
C The patient will be unable to stand on tip-toe
D Surgical repair may be complicated by wound breakdown
E No treatment is necessary in the elderly patient

Answers

232 A **False** B **True** C **False** D **True** E **False**

Fractures through the neck of the humerus require two radiographs, an antero-posterior and lateral, to define the degree of displacement. A single view may give misleading information. Complications of the fracture include damage to the axillary nerve as it winds around the neck of the humerus to supply the deltoid muscle and an area of skin over the muscle. Severe displacement may result in a brachial plexus injury. Avascular necrosis of the head of the humerus is a rare complication whereas shoulder stiffness, especially in older patients, is frequent. Conservative treatment is indicated in most fractures with support by a broad arm sling since providing there is good apposition of the bone ends, non-union is uncommon. Occasionally a manipulation under anaesthetic is necessary to produce a good alignment of the fragments.

233 A **False** B **True** C **True** D **True** E **False**

Most ruptures of the tendo achillis occur in adults, either spontaneously or, occasionally, after steroid injections into the tendon. If the rupture is left untreated, the tendon will unite with lengthening. As a result, running and jumping will be difficult due to weakness of plantarflexion of the ankle. Conservative treatment by plaster with the ankle in equinus for a period of about 8 weeks should be advised in the older age group to decrease morbidity. Operative repair is probably advisable in younger athletic individuals to decrease the risk of tendon lengthening. One of the dangers of operative repair is wound breakdown which may endanger the tendon repair and require skin grafting.

Questions (*Answers overleaf*)

234 In children, fractures of the lateral condyle of the humerus

- **A** may be confused with normal epiphyseal lines when they are undisplaced
- **B** may be missed because the condyle is mainly cartilaginous in young children
- **C** may result in non-union when displaced fractures are treated conservatively without accurate reduction
- **D** usually involve the whole of the trochlea and half of the capitellum
- **E** should be treated by open reduction and Kirschner wire fixation if closed methods fail to reduce the fracture

235 In posterior dislocation of the shoulder

- **A** if the dislocation is unstable after reduction, a shoulder spica holding the humerus abducted 40° and externally rotated may be necessary
- **B** habitual dislocations are often associated with psychiatric problems
- **C** recurrent dislocation following treatment is a recognised complication
- **D** diagnosis can easily be made on routine radiographs
- **E** axillary nerve injury is common

Answers

234 A **True** B **True** C **True** D **False** E **True**

A fall on the outstretched hand may result in the force being transmitted through the radius against the lateral condyle of the humerus. Usually the fracture includes the capitellum and half of the trochlea. Radiographs should be carefully examined especially in small children since the lower end of the humerus is mainly cartilaginous. If doubt exists, radiographs of the opposite elbow should be obtained for comparison. Completely displaced fractures should be treated by accurate reduction and fixation of the intra-articular fracture to decrease the well recognised risk of non-union. Minimally displaced fractures may be reduced and treated conservatively with the elbow flexed, providing serial radiographs are taken to ensure that the reduction is maintained.

235 A **True** B **True** C **True** D **False** E **False**

Posterior dislocation of the shoulder is notorious for being missed on initial examination. The displacement following the injury is not as marked as an anterior dislocation. An antero-posterior radiograph may not show an obvious dislocation. A high index of suspicion, careful clinical examination to demonstrate restricted external rotation and a lateral radiograph of the shoulder are necessary to confirm the diagnosis. Reduction by manipulation under anaesthetic may be unstable requiring a plaster spica for shoulder immobilisation from 4–6 weeks. Habitual dislocation of the shoulder is associated with a psychiatric disorder in some patients. In contrast to anterior dislocation, injury to the axillary nerve is rare.

Questions (*Answers overleaf*)

236 Fractures of the radial head
- **A** may be associated with inferior radio-ulnar subluxation
- **B** are commoner in children than adults
- **C** can be treated by rest in a broad arm sling for 3 weeks if undisplaced
- **D** may require immediate excision of the radial head when displaced and comminuted
- **E** may result in permanent loss of full extension of the elbow

237 In dislocations of the elbow
- **A** an anterior dislocation is more common than a posterior dislocation
- **B** the medial epicondyle may be pulled off and may be retained in the joint after reduction of the dislocation
- **C** myositis ossificans is a well recognised complication
- **D** an anterior dislocation is associated with a fracture of the proximal radius
- **E** recurrent dislocation is common despite expert treatment

Answers

236 A **True** B **False** C **True** D **True** E **True**

Fractures of the radial head tend to occur in adults whereas a fracture of the neck of the radius is seen in children. Undisplaced fractures may be treated by rest for about 3 weeks in a broad arm sling followed by active elbow exercises. A severe injury with displacement of the radial head may result in rupture of the interosseous ligament and subluxation of the distal radio-ulnar joint due to proximal migration of the radius. Severe displaced fractures are treated by immediate excision of all the fragments or delayed excision about 2 months from injury. Some surgeons replace the radial head with a silastic prosthesis to maintain the length of the radius. Even in minor injuries to the radial head permanent restricted elbow movements may complicate recovery.

237 A **False** B **True** C **True** D **False** E **False**

Most dislocations of the elbow are postero-lateral. Occasionally the dislocation is anterior when the radial head dislocates and the ulna fractures, in the olecranon fossa. Complications include myositis ossificans and joint stiffness, often said to be related to early passive mobilisation. In children, the medial epicondyle may be pulled off and retained in the elbow joint following reduction of the dislocation. The fragment must be removed to avoid restricted elbow movement and the development of secondary osteoarthritis. Recurrent dislocation is uncommon and is associated with disorders such as Ehlers Danlos syndrome or familial joint laxity.

Questions (*Answers overleaf*)

238 Olecranon fractures

A can be mistaken for normal epiphyseal lines in children
B are frequently avulsion fractures
C may be associated with anterior dislocation of the elbow
D usually require open reduction and internal fixation when displaced, to maintain congruity of the joint and to restore the extensor mechanism of the elbow
E may be treated conservatively in an above-elbow plaster if undisplaced, for a period of 6–8 weeks in an adult

239 Fractures of the neck of the radius in children

A are less common than radial head fractures
B usually occur through the proximal radial epiphysis
C should be treated by immediate excision of the radial head when markedly displaced
D are usually caused by a fall on the outstretched hand
E may be reduced by gentle manipulation by pronation and supination of the forearm where the head is tilted less than 30° to the long axis of the radius

240 Complications of a fracture of the middle third of the radius and ulna treated by plate fixation include

A non-union
B restriction of pronation and supination
C cross-union
D infection
E damage to the ulnar nerve in proximal radial fractures

Answers

238 A **True** B **True** C **True** D **True** E **True**

The olecranon may be fractured by a direct injury to the point of the elbow or by a sudden pull of the triceps producing an avulsion fracture. A lateral radiograph will confirm the fracture, but occasionally the proximal ulnar epiphysis may be mistaken for an undisplaced fracture in children. Radiographs of the opposite uninjured elbow will clarify the situation. Treatment of undisplaced fractures is by broad arm sling or plaster until the fracture has healed, about 6–8 weeks from injury. Serial radiographs are essential to ensure the fracture does not displace. Displaced fractures usually require open reduction and fixation by a screw or tension band to restore continuity of the joint surface and to restore the extensor mechanism. An anterior dislocation of the elbow is associated with a fracture of the olecranon and a dislocation of the radial head.

239 A **False** B **True** C **False** D **True** E **True**

Whereas fractures of the head of the radius tend to occur in adults, fractures of the neck of the radius occur in children through the proximal radial epiphyseal plate (Salter Type II epiphyseal injury). The fracture is usually caused by a fall on the outstretched hand. If angulation persists, gentle manipulation of the radial head may be performed. Severe angulation may require open reduction and fixation of the radial head by a Kirschner wire. The radial head should never be excised in children since this will result in subluxation of the distal radio-ulnar joint.

240 A **True** B **True** C **True** D **True** E **False**

Displaced midshaft fractures of the radius and ulna are frequently treated by plate fixation to maintain alignment and restore length. As in any operation, infection may complicate postoperative progress. The posterior interosseous nerve may be injured at operation especially where dissection around the proximal part of the radius is necessary, since the nerve is vulnerable as it passes round the neck of the radius. Cross-union of the radius and ulna is a well known complication of internal fixation and results in restriction of pronation and supination. Non-union is another well recognised complication, possibly due to excessive stripping of the periosteum from the bone ends.

Questions (*Answers overleaf*)

241 Following a fracture of the medial epicondyle of the elbow in children

A even with slight displacement, the epicondyle should be reduced and treated by internal fixation to reduce the risk of medial ligament laxity
B care should be taken when interpreting radiographs to ensure the fragment does not lie within the elbow joint
C there may occasionally be an ulnar nerve palsy
D flexor muscle strength in the forearm is permanently weakened
E there may be permanent stiffness of the elbow joint

242 Which of the following are features of the acute central cord syndrome

A A fracture-dislocation at the mid-cervical spine
B A hyperextension injury to the cervical spine in the presence of cervical spondylosis
C The prognosis for recovery is better in the upper than the lower limbs
D Bladder function does not usually return
E There is a lower motor neurone lesion in the upper limbs and an upper motor neurone lesion in the lower limbs

Answers

241 A **False**
B **True**
C **True**
D **False**
E **True**

Fractures of the medial epicondyle usually result in a mild displacement of the fragment. Occasionally, after dislocation of the elbow, the medial epicondyle may displace into the elbow joint. Besides dislocation, other mechanisms of injury include abduction of the elbow resulting in a 'pull off' fracture where the ulnar collateral ligament inserts, sudden contraction of the flexor muscle mass or by direct injury. Treatment is usually symptomatic for relatively undisplaced fractures, but a markedly displaced fracture or one with the fragment in the elbow joint requires open reduction and internal fixation by a Kirschner wire. Occasionally there may be an ulnar nerve lesion but this is nearly always a lesion in continuity and will recover. As with all fractures around the elbow, there is a possibility of permanent joint stiffness. Flexor weakness is minimal or absent, presumably due to the wide muscular origin.

242 A **False**
B **True**
C **False**
D **False**
E **True**

The acute central cord syndrome usually occurs after a hyperextension injury to the cervical spine in which there is cervical spondylosis or some other disorder in which there are localised areas of fusion. The resultant neurological picture appears to be related to cord ischaemia caused by damage to the spinal vessels which may be transient or permanent. Motor weakness is usually upper motor neurone in the lower limbs and lower motor in the upper limbs. Initially, there may be urinary retention which usually recovers later. Temperature and pain sensitivity are more effected than proprioception and light touch. Prognosis is often good, especially in the lower limbs. Fine hand movements (TI) frequently fail to recover. Treatment is by resting the cervical spine in a well-fitting collar together with intensive physiotherapy to the limbs.

Questions (*Answers overleaf*)

243 In a unifacet dislocation of the cervical spine

- **A** the mechanism of injury is flexion and rotation
- **B** the lateral radiograph will show a displacement of one vertebral body on the other by a third of the diameter of the body
- **C** the dislocation may be reduced by gentle manipulation of the spine under general anaesthetic if expert supervision is available
- **D** skull traction may be applied with increasing weight and serial radiographs until the dislocation is reduced
- **E** there is invariably transection of the cord at the level of injury

244 Following reduction of fractures of the midshaft of tibia

- **A** an internal rotation deformity of 15° distal to the fracture is acceptable
- **B** varus bowing of the tibia is cosmetically more acceptable than valgus
- **C** valgus bowing of the tibia is cosmetically more acceptable than varus
- **D** external rotation of the distal fragment on the proximal by 15° results in difficulty in walking
- **E** a laterally based opening plaster wedge may be used to reduce a valgus angulation at the fracture site

Answers

243 A **True**
B **True**
C **True**
D **True**
E **False**

A unifacet dislocation of the spine is caused by a flexion and rotation injury. The patient complains of neck pain and inability to straighten the neck. The patient may or may not have a transected cord, depending on the effect of violence on the spinal cord. Diagnosis is confirmed by radiographs of the spine including lateral and oblique views. At the site of the dislocation, the body of one vertebra will be subluxed forward on the other by about a third of a body diameter. Reduction of the dislocation is by either gentle manipulation under anaesthetic or by skull traction with increasing weights and repeated radiographs while the patient is awake to carefully monitor any change in neurology.

244 A **False**
B **True**
C **False**
D **False**
E **True**

Alignment of tibial fractures should be as near anatomical as possible. Persistent varus-valgus angulation may result in abnormal stress on the ankle or knee joint resulting in pain and degenerative change. In women even minor degrees of valgus angulation may produce a bony prominence under the subcutaneous border of the tibia which is unsightly. A similar varus angulation may be unnoticeable. An external rotation deformity of 15° may be acceptable in regard to normal gait, whereas a similar internal rotation deformity will result in a poor gait because the foot will tend to catch on the ground. Following manipulation of the fracture and application of a plaster, angulation may be reduced by opening wedges in the plaster which are held open by a prepared piece of cork. It is important to remember that rotational alignment of the fracture can only be judged clinically and not from radiographs.

Questions (*Answers overleaf*)

245 Osteochondral fractures of the femoral condyle
- **A** may be associated with lateral dislocation of the patella
- **B** are easily missed on radiographic examination because the fragment consists mainly of cartilage
- **C** may require exploration of the knee joint with replacement of a large fragment and fixation by a Smillie pin
- **D** small fragments may be removed and the defect allowed to fill with fibrocartilage
- **E** may result in symptoms of giving way

246 Pathological long bone fractures associated with malignant disease
- **A** most commonly occur in breast carcinoma
- **B** most frequently affect the femur and humerus
- **C** should be treated by conservative means if possible
- **D** may be a presenting feature of malignancy
- **E** invariably unite providing the fracture can be adequately immobilised

247 A posterior cruciate tear of the knee
- **A** may be caused by a blow from a dashboard on the tibial tubercle with the knee flexed
- **B** may be identified by the tibia sagging backward on the femur with the knee flexed
- **C** may be confirmed by an avulsed fragment of bone in the anterior part of the tibial spines on the lateral view radiograph
- **D** will be associated with a haemarthrosis in the acute stage
- **E** may be repaired by a medial parapatellar incision in the knee joint

Answers

245 A **True** B **True** C **True** D **True** E **True**

Osteochondral fractures within the knee joint are not uncommon. They are associated with dislocation of the patella, which shears off part of the lateral femoral condyle. Flakes of the patella may also be sheared off. Direct injury to the knee may also produce the fractures. Fragments are easily missed on radiographs, either because they are small or mainly cartilaginous. Large fragments should be replaced and fixed with Smillie pins, while small fragments may be removed. If fragments remain in the knee joint, they may continue to grow and act as loose bodies resulting in symptoms of giving way, locking and pain.

246 A **True** B **True** C **False** D **True** E **False**

Pathological fractures from malignant disease most frequently occur in carcinoma of the breast. The other common tumours are thyroid, lung, prostate and kidney. Occasionally the original site is unknown and the fracture is the presenting feature of malignancy. The site of the fracture is most commonly the upper end of femur and less commonly in the humerus and tibia. The aim of treatment is to immobilise the fracture to relieve pain and improve function and also to arrest expansion of the tumour by chemotherapy or radiotherapy. The optimal method is by internal fixation, occasionally using methyl methacrylate cement if bone is missing. The fractures may unite normally, but others continue to produce bone lysis unless treated by radiotherapy or other means.

247 A **True** B **True** C **False** D **True** E **False**

The posterior cruciate ligament is usually ruptured or avulsed from its insertion into the posterior edge of the tibial eminence by an injury which pushes the tibia backwards on the femur with the knee flexed. On examination, there will be a haemarthrosis and the tibia will sag back on the femur when the patient lies supine with both hip and knees flexed and the examiner holding the heel. Routine radiographs will show either no abnormality or an avulsion fracture of the posterior edge of the tibial plateau. Any operative repair must be from the back of the knee since the posterior cruciate is hidden from view anteriorly by bony structures and the anterior cruciate.

Questions (*Answers overleaf*)

248 Rupture of the lateral structures of the knee in a young footballer

A may be associated with a complete common peroneal nerve palsy
B occasionally results in a fracture of the tip of the fibula head, identified on radiographs
C may require stress radiographs to confirm diagnosis
D usually requires treatment by plaster cylinder for 6 weeks
E may include rupture of the lateral ligament, capsule, and biceps femoris

249 Pellegrini-Stieda's disease

A occurs after a varus strain of the knee resulting in a partial avulsion of the femoral origin of the lateral ligament
B presents on radiographic examination as an area of calcification over the medial femoral condyle
C requires open reduction and repair of the collateral ligament
D may be treated by a hydrocortisone injection
E may be an incidental finding on routine radiographs

250 Fractures of the lateral tibial plateau

A are usually caused by a valgus force on the knee
B are usually caused by a varus force on the knee
C may be associated with medial ligament rupture in severe cases
D are less common than fractures of the medial plateau
E may require tomograms of the knee to define the amount of depression of the tibial plateau

Answers

248 A **True** B **True** C **True** D **False** E **True**

The lateral structures including the lateral ligament, biceps femoris and the lateral capsule may be torn by a force on the inner side of the knee. If severe, there may be a traction injury to the common peroneal nerve. Radiographs may show no abnormality or a fracture of the head of the fibula where the lateral ligament has been avulsed or from the tibia where the antero-lateral capsule has been pulled off. Stress views will demonstrate the degree of varus instability. A complete ligament and capsular rupture requires an open operation to repair the structures, especially the postero-lateral capsule. A plaster is applied for a period of about 6 weeks with the knee flexed to 30°.

249 A **False** B **True** C **False** D **True** E **True**

A partial rupture or avulsion of the medial ligament from its insertion on the medial condyle may result in calcification. The patient will complain of persistent aching pain and stiffness in the knee. On examination there will be localised tenderness and perhaps pain on straining the knee in valgus with slight flexion. Radiographs will demonstrate the area of calcification. Treatment includes either a period of rest in plaster or a hydrocortisone injection into the tender spot. Frequently the area of calcification fails to disappear despite the fact that symptoms may settle.

250 A **True** B **False** C **True** D **False** E **True**

Lateral tibial plateau fractures usually occur when the knee is struck on the lateral side and the femoral condyle is crushed into the lateral tibial plateau. Usually the force of the impact is absorbed by the fracture, but occasionally the injury may be severe enough to rupture the medial ligament. Lateral plateau fractures are more common than medial, since to some extent, the inner side of the leg is protected from direct injury by the opposite leg. Frequently tomograms will demonstrate that the amount of plateau depression is much greater than realised on the original routine radiographs.

Questions (*Answers overleaf*)

251 Complications of closed midshaft fractures of the femur include

A fat embolism
B mal-union
C delayed union
D femoral nerve palsy
E hypovolaemic shock

252 Displaced fractures of the supracondylar region of the femur

A may be treated by an intramedullary Kuntscher nail
B usually result in anterior tilt of the distal fragment
C usually result in posterior tilt of the distal fragment
D Can usually be reduced and treated with the knee extended in a Thomas splint
E may be associated with rupture of the popliteal artery

Answers

251 A **True** Fractures of the femur may be complicated by both local and generalised problems
B **True**
C **True**
D **False**
E **True**

Local: Mal-union — shortening
— angulation
— rotation
Delayed union or non-union — idiopathic
— high velocity injury
— soft tissue interposition.

General: Hypovolaemic shock — Bone and soft tissue injury (often 1–1½ litre blood loss)
Fat embolus
Pneumonia
Deep venous thrombosis
Pulmonary embolism
Bed sores — due to prolonged immobilization.

Nerve palsies are uncommon in femoral fractures presumably due to the protective layers of muscle between nerve and bone. Femoral nerve palsy is highly unlikely since the nerve has innervated its muscle by the time it has reached the midshaft region of the femur.

252 A **False** Displaced supracondylar fractures result in rotation of the distal fragment backwards due to the pull of the gastrocnemius at its insertion into the posterior aspect of the condyles. This problem may be overcome at the time of reduction by flexing the knee. The bony spikes at the site of the fracture which angulate backwards, may pierce the popliteal artery causing ischaemia of the limb. Careful observation of the circulation distal to the fracture is mandatory. Treatment may be conservative using a Thomas splint with a Pearson knee flexion piece or by open reduction and internal fixation using a blade-plate. An intramedullary nail is unlikely to hold the fracture.
B **True**
C **False**
D **False**
E **True**

Questions (*Answers overleaf*)

253 In the anatomy of the spinal cord

A the spinal cord ends at the level of the third lumbar vertebra

B the spinal cord ends at the level of the first lumbar vertebra

C the lumbar and sacral nerve root segments of the cord lie between the 10th thoracic and first lumbar vertebrae

D the seventh cervical nerve root passes out through the foramen between the seventh cervical and first thoracic vertebra

E the posterior columns contain fibres for proprioception, touch, vibration and pressure sensation

254 Concerning spinal cord injury

A Return of the reflex activity with absence of sensation and voluntary muscle activity confirms a good prognosis

B Partial sensory sparing and muscle activity 12 hours after injury confirms that complete transection has not occured

C A complete absence of neurological activity below the site of injury at initial examination confirms that the spinal cord has been transected

D A lesion of the cauda equina presents with lower motor neurone signs

E A partial lesion at the thoraco-lumbar junction may produce both upper and lower motor neurone signs

Answers

253 A **False** B **True** C **True** D **False** E **True**

The spinal cord ends at the level of the first lumbar vertebra. Distal to this point the nerve roots (cauda equina) fill the spinal canal. All the lumbar and sacral nerve root segments arise from the cord at the level of the tenth thoracic and first lumbar vertebrae and pass down the canal before exiting through their vertebral foramina. It should be remembered that there are seven cervical vertebrae with eight cervical nerve roots. The first to seventh cervical roots pass out above their respective vertebrae, while the eighth passes out below the seventh cervical vertebra.

254 A **False** B **True** C **False** D **True** E **True**

Immediately following spinal cord injury, spinal concussion' may be demonstrated by a patchy distribution or complete absence of neurological signs distal to the injury. With an intact spinal cord, some neurological improvement will occur within the next 24–48 hours. In a complete transection, the reflexes will return without controlled motor function or return of sensation. A lesion at the level of the cauda equina will present as a lower motor neurone lesion since there is involvement of only peripheral nerves at this level. At the thoraco-lumbar junction both the lumbar spinal cord segments and part of the cauda equina are present. Injury at this level may produce a mixed picture with upper motor neurone signs due to spontaneous reflex activity distal to the cord damage and also lower motor neurone signs due to damage to the peripheral nerves of the cauda equina.

Questions (*Answers overleaf*)

255 Following a fracture

- **A** there is death of bone cells adjacent to the fracture
- **B** woven bone is formed beneath the periosteum which bridges the fracture fragments
- **C** excessive mobility at the fracture site may disrupt the bridging callus
- **D** cells within the medullary cavity take no part in fracture healing
- **E** cortical bone and its cellular constituents take no part in fracture healing despite apposition of the bone ends

256 Concerning displaced intra-articular fractures in the lower limb, in young adults

- **A** Early open reduction and internal fixation may reduce the risk of secondary osteoarthritis
- **B** Joint stiffness may result from extra and intra-articular adhesions
- **C** A fracture through the lateral condyle of the femur frequently results in avascular necrosis
- **D** Joint stiffness will be decreased by delayed mobilisation of the joint
- **E** Non-union of tibial plateau fractures is a frequent complication

Answers

255 A **True** B **True** C **True** D **False** E **False**

Following a fracture, the periosteum is stripped from the cortex and there is haemorrhage into the fracture gap. There is bone necrosis to a lesser or greater degree at the fracture site. New bone may develop from each of these three sites; periosteum, medulla and bone cortex. The periosteum produces new woven bone which creeps across from each side of the fracture to join, forming a bridge of callus. The medullary haematoma becomes infiltrated with blood vessels and fibrous tissue and subsequently calcium salts are deposited to form bone. If the cortical bone ends are apposed and subject to very little movement, blood vessels grow across the bone ends revitalising the dead area and lay down new bone; primary bone healing. In the first two methods of fracture healing, the woven immature bone is replaced by new Haversian systems along the lines of stress until the architecture is fully reconstituted.

256 A **True** B **True** C **False** D **False** E **False**

Intra-articular fractures of the lower limb are serious injuries associated with the complications of joint stiffness and secondary osteoarthritis. Avascular necrosis of the femoral condyle is a very rare complication, probably because the blood supply is good and the fracture is mainly through cancellous bone. Non-union of a tibial plateau fracture is again rare unless there is wide separation of the fragments. Accurate reduction and its maintainance is essential to decrease the risk of arthritis in intra-articular fractures. Internal fixation may allow early mobilisation, reducing the risk of joint stiffness.

Questions (*Answers overleaf*)

257 A Smith's fracture
- **A** occurs at the distal end of the radius
- **B** results in dorsal tilt and displacement of the distal fragment
- **C** usually requires a lateral radiograph of the wrist to differentiate it from a Colles' fracture
- **D** can usually be treated in a Colles-type plaster after reduction
- **E** usually requires 12 weeks immobilisation before union occurs

258 A Colles' fracture
- **A** occurs in the radius about 1 inch proximal to the wrist and is associated with a fracture of the ulnar styloid
- **B** is usually associated with ulnar displacement together with dorsal displacement and tilting of the distal fragment
- **C** was described by an English surgeon in the nineteenth century
- **D** often results in a fracture of the ulnar styloid, since the distal displaced radial fragment is attached to the ulna by the triangular cartilage
- **E** is frequently seen in the elderly patient, where osteoporosis is a predisposing factor

259 A displaced T–Y fracture of the lower end of the femur in a 25 year old male
- **A** can be easily managed by skeletal traction
- **B** should be accurately reduced and fixed with a blade plate and screws
- **C** may be complicated by stiffness of movements in the knee joint despite accurate reduction
- **D** frequently results in non-union despite accurate reduction
- **E** may be immobilised in a plaster of paris cylinder and the patient allowed to weight-bear

Answers

257 A **True** B **False** C **True** D **False** E **False**

A Smith's fracture, much rarer than a Colles' fracture at the wrist, occurs at the distal half to an inch of the radius with palmar tilt and palmar displacement of the distal fragment. Unless a lateral view of the wrist is seen on radiographs, then the fracture may be mistaken for a Colles' fracture on the antero-posterior film. The fracture is often easy to reduce under general anaesthetic, but difficult to hold until union using a Colles-type plaster. A superior way to hold reduction is by supinating the forearm and holding the fracture with the wrist slightly dorsiflexed in an above-elbow plaster for a period of about 6 weeks.

258 A **True** B **False** C **False** D **True** E **True**

Colles' fracture was originally described in 1814 by Abraham Colles, a surgeon from Ireland. It is a fracture at the distal inch of the radius, and when displaced results in radial deviation, dorsal tilt and dorsal displacement of the distal fragment producing the classical 'dinner fork' deformity. Because the tri-radiate fibro-cartilage is attached to the distal fragment of the radius, displacement results in a pull-off of the ulnar styloid. The fracture is commonly seen in osteoporotic forearms of the elderly but is also seen in the young following more severe trauma.

259 A **False** B **True** C **True** D **False** E **False**

A displaced T–Y fracture of the lower end of the femur is a serious injury requiring accurate reduction and internal fixation. By this method of treatment the articular surface will be restored, possibly decreasing the risk of secondary arthritis and allowing early movement reducing the risk of knee stiffness. Non-union of these fractures is uncommon, possibly because of good blood supply and abundant cancellous bone.

Questions (*Answers overleaf*)

260 An avulsion fracture of the anterior tibial spine in a 20 year old male

A should be treated by excision of the fragment to allow a full range of knee flexion
B should be accurately reduced and fixed by a screw
C should be treated by early mobilisation disregarding the fracture
D may be treated in an above-knee plaster with slight knee flexion providing radiographs show accurate reduction of the fracture
E always carries a good prognosis despite the lack of treatment

261 Factors associated with delayed or non-union of a fracture are

A A low velocity type of injury
B Soft-tissue interposition between the fragments
C The presence of large areas of cancellous bone
D Excessive movement at the fracture site
E Interruption of the blood supply to the bone fragments

Answers

260 A **False** B **True** C **False** D **True** E **False**

An avulsion fracture of the tibial spine usually occurs after a hyperextension injury of the knee or following a twisting injury in which instead of the anterior cruciate breaking, the bony insertion is pulled out of the tibia. Careful examination of the radiographs of the knee are essential for diagnosis. Undisplaced fractures may be treated conservatively in a plaster cylinder with slight knee flexion. Displaced fractures should be opened and the fragment screwed back into position in order to restore the function of the anterior cruciate. Reduction will also prevent the fragment causing reduction of movement due to impingement on the femoral condyles.

261 A **False** B **True** C **False** D **True** E **True**

Excessive mobility at a fracture site is a cause of non-union since it results in breakdown of periosteal bridging callus, and endosteal callus. This type of non-union frequently results in hypertrophic non-union with abundant callus formation. Treatment is by fixation of the fracture to decrease movement. Soft-tissue interposition or over distraction results in failure of bridging callus across the fracture fragments. High velocity injuries are more likely to result in non-union due to bone death, stripping of periosteum and soft tissues. Poor blood supply may be a cause of non-union, but equally avascular necrosis of the proximal pole of the scaphoid and femoral head may still go on to union by creeping substitution. Cancellous bone has a greater potential to form fracture callus compared to cortical bone.

Questions (*Answers overleaf*)

262 A patient of 22 years presents with a history of giving way of the ankle. A diagnosis of chronic rupture of the lateral ligament of the ankle is suspected

- **A** Routine radiographs of the ankle are usually normal
- **B** Inversion stress views of the ankle under general anaesthetic would confirm the diagnosis
- **C** The ankle should be treated in a below-knee plaster of paris for 6 weeks
- **D** An alternative diagnosis may be a loose body within the ankle joint
- **E** Reinforcement of the lateral ligament by the tendon of peroneus brevis is an accepted method of treatment when the diagnosis is confirmed

263 In dislocations of the lunate

- **A** the dislocation is seen most easily on the antero-posterior radiograph
- **B** the capitate is aligned with the lunate on the lateral radiograph
- **C** The capitate is aligned with the radius on the lateral radiograph
- **D** despite reduction, avascular necrosis of the lunate is a known complication
- **E** the patient may develop symptoms of acute median nerve compression

Answers

262 A **True** B **True** C **False** D **True** E **True**

A chronic rupture of the lateral ligament of the ankle presents with a history of recurrent giving way and ankle swelling. In between attacks of pain and giving way, signs may be minimal apart from a suggestion of increased laxity on inversion of the ankle. Routine radiographs are usually normal, though occasionally an ununited avulsion fracture of the tip of the lateral malleolus may be present. Stress views under general anaesthetic would confirm diagnosis showing increased varus tilt and anterior subluxation of the talus in the ankle mortice. Conservative treatment is of little value in chronic cases, apart from an outer flapper to the heel. Reinforcement of the ligament by routing peroneus brevis through the distal end of the fibula usually reduces the symptoms of giving way. Loose bodies are another cause of giving way of the ankle.

263 A **False** B **False** C **True** D **True** E **True**

Lunate dislocations are usually the final stage of perilunar dislocations of the carpus. Following a fall on the outstretched hand, the capitate dislocates posteriorly off the lunate. Due to elasticity within the intact ligaments, the capitate re-alignes itself with the radius pushing the lunate volar-wards and rotated by 90°. Pressure of the lunate on the median nerve within the carpal tunnel may result in acute carpal tunnel syndrome. A lateral radiograph is most useful in these injuries. Normally the three C's of radius, lunate and capitate are aligned. In a dislocation of the lunate, the C′ of the radius is aligned with the C′ of the capitate, with the lunate lying in a volar position. Due to damage to the blood supply of the lunate, it may become avascular.

Questions (*Answers overleaf*)

264 Concerning closed midshaft fractures of the proximal phalanges of the hand

A A transverse fracture usually results in palmar tilt at the fracture site
B A transverse fracture is usually stable when the fracture is reduced and the finger flexed
C Rotational deformity following reduction can be easily identified on post-reduction radiographs
D Residual stiffness of the proximal interphalangeal joint is very uncommon
E Unstable oblique fractures may require fixation by Kirshner wire to maintain reduction

265 Concerning remodelling of a fracture of the tibia in a child aged between 6 years and 12 years

A Rotational deformity would be expected to remodel completely
B Varus-valgus angulation would be expected to improve
C The older the child, the greater the potential for remodelling
D The nearer the deformity to a joint, the less likely is remodelling to occur
E Deformity in the plane of the adjacent joint is likely to improve

266 Traumatic displacement of the lower femoral epiphysis

A is usually associated with posterior displacement of the distal fragment
B is usually caused by a hyperextension injury to the knee
C may result in damage to the popliteal artery
D rarely results in premature fusion of the epiphysis
E frequently results in knee stiffness despite treatment

Answers

264 A **False**
B **True**
C **False**
D **False**
E **True**

Fractures through the proximal phalanx of the finger require careful management since residual deformity may greatly compromise hand function. Despite good management, joint stiffness at the proximal interphalangeal joint and adhesions of the extensor hood to the fracture may compromise final function. Transverse fractures tilt dorsally due to intrinsic pull and are usually stable with flexion of the finger over a splint. Oblique fractures which are unstable usually require internal fixation to maintain length and avoid angulation. Rotational deformity is difficult to identify on radiographs and should be assessed clinically by comparing the position of the tip of the injured finger with adjacent digits.

265 A **False**
B **True**
C **False**
D **False**
E **True**

The potential for remodelling of a fracture is most impressive in children and is related to age; the younger the child, the greater potential. However, remodelling of an axial rotational deformity is poor. In comparison, where there is angulation in the plane of an adjacent joint, varus or valgus angulation or where the deformity is near to the joint and epiphyseal plate, there is a good potential for remodelling. It should be emphasised that the potential for remodelling should not be an excuse for poor reduction of a fracture, since its effect is variable and may not resolve gross deformity.

266 A **False**
B **True**
C **True**
D **True**
E **False**

Traumatic displacement of the lower femoral epiphysis is usually associated with a hyperextension injury to the knee resulting in anterior displacement of the distal fragment. Compromise of the popliteal vessels by external pressure or by direct injury may result in limb ischaemia. Early reduction is essential to reduce this risk. Delay in treatment after 24–48 hours may result in difficulty in reduction since the fragments may already be firmly adherent to each other. Premature fusion is uncommon and knee movement usually returns completely in uncomplicated cases.

Questions (*Answers overleaf*)

267 Concerning closed fractures of the shaft of the femur in an adult

A An intramedullary Kuntscher nail can be used to hold an oblique fracture of the lower third
B An intramedullary Kuntscher nail can be used to hold a transverse midshaft fracture
C Lower third fractures may be held with a blade-plate
D A cast-brace is an alternative to internal fixation in fractures of the lower and middle thirds
E Internal fixation is contra-indicated in patients with prolonged unconsciousness, or restlessness from head injury

268 In rupture of the patellar ligament

A the knee cannot be actively extended
B radiographs will show an abnormal position of the patella
C a palpable gap may be found between the tibial tuberosity and the patella
D conservative treatment is advised
E there may be a bone fragment attached to the distal end of the patellar ligament

269 Complete laceration of the common peroneal nerve at the neck of the fibula will result in

A weakness of eversion of the foot
B inability to invert the foot
C loss of activity in the extensor hallucis and extensor digitorum longus
D normal sensation in the affected foot
E normal power of plantarflexion of the foot

Answers

267 A **False** B **True** C **True** D **True** E **False**

Intramedullary Kuntscher nailing is ideal in the segment of the femur in which the medullary canal is narrowest and where the fracture is transverse and will be stable to compression after fixation. It would be unsuitable in distal oblique fractures since the medullary canal is widening and compression stability would not be obtained. A blade-plate should be used in lower third fractures rather than a nail. A cast-brace is a useful alternative to internal fixation of lower third fractures since it will hold the reduced fracture and allow knee flexion. In patients with prolonged unconsciousness and restlessness, internal fixation of fractures should be the rule to allow ease of nursing and maintenance of a satisfactory reduction of the fracture.

268 A **True** B **True** C **True** D **False** E **True**

Rupture of the patellar ligament usually occurs after sudden resistance to forceful extension of the knee. The ligament may be avulsed from the lower pole of the patella or the tibial tuberosity, perhaps with a fragment of bone, or ruptured in the substance of the ligament. The diagnosis depends on clinical examination. There will be tenderness over the ligament, perhaps a palpable gap and elevation of the patella. A lateral radiograph will show a more proximal position of the patella compared to the normal side. The patient will not be able to actively extend the knee. Treatment is by operative repair of the ligament and immobilisation in a plaster cylinder for about 6 weeks.

269 A **True** B **False** C **True** D **False** E **True**

The common peroneal nerve divides into the deep peroneal nerve and the superficial peroneal nerve. The former supplies the extensor digitorium longus; tibialis anterior; extensor hallucis longus; peroneus tertius; extensor digitorum brevis; and supplies skin of the first interdigital cleft. The superficial peroneal nerve supplies the peroneal muscles and skin over the peronei and extensor muscles in the distal half of the leg. Other cutaneous branches include the sural communicating nerve to the skin of the lateral side of the little toe and the lateral cutaneous nerve of the calf which supplies skin over the upper half of the lateral side of the calf.

Questions (*Answers overleaf*)

270 Following a clean laceration to the flexor tendons of the index finger

A repair of the tendons in the palm carries a better prognosis than a similar injury at the level of the proximal phalanx

B delayed tendon grafting should be considered for a laceration at the level of the proximal phalanx if the surgeon is inexperienced

C a laceration distal to the terminal interphalangeal joint carries a better prognosis than one at the proximal joint

D the palmaris longus tendon should not be used as a tendon graft in the finger

E tenolysis should be delayed for at least 6 months following primary repair of the tendons in which adhesions have developed

271 A 20 year old male sustains a closed displaced oblique fracture of the tibia treated initially by closed reduction and application of above knee plaster. The fracture redisplaces after one week with approximately 2″ of shortening

A The fracture should be remanipulated and a further plaster applied

B The plaster may be wedged

C The position should be accepted

D Open reduction and internal fixation of the tibia would be an accepted form of treatment

E A pin may be placed in the lower tibia and the fracture held out to length by traction and angulation treated by plaster

Answers

270 A **True** B **True** C **True** D **False** E **True**

Clean lacerations to the flexor tendons of the finger require expert management. Adhesions and failure of healing are common complications and may result in a useless finger. Lacerations distal to the terminal interphalangeal joint carry a good prognosis since only one tendon, the profundus, is involved. In the palm, repair of tendons usually produces good results since there is space available and adhesions that may form do not usually result in serious restriction of movement. The problem area lies between the distal palmar crease and the insertion of the sublimis into the middle phalanx. Here, two tendons lie within a rigid fibrous flexor sheath with restricted volume. This factor may result in poor excursion of the repaired tendons from both bulk and adhesions. An alternative to primary repair is a delayed tendon graft using a palmaris longus tendon, though results are not always satisfactory. If the repair becomes firmly fixed to adjacent structures by adhesions, an attempt to release the repair should be delayed for at least 6 months otherwise adhesions will rapidly reform.

271 A **False** B **False** C **False** D **True** E **True**

Oblique displaced fractures of the tibia are difficult to hold by simple plaster fixation. They tend to collapse with shortening. A loss of length of two inches is not acceptable. The fracture may be held out to length by internal fixation raising the problems of skin necrosis and infection. An alternative method of treatment is by pin traction and plaster immobilisation or by inserting pins above and below the fracture and incorporating the pins in plaster. This latter method may be useful where skin cover is potentially at risk. A re-manipulation and application of plaster will probably result in further loss of reduction.

Questions (*Answers overleaf*)

272 In non-union of the scaphoid

- **A** the patient may remain asymptomatic
- **B** osteoarthritis of the radio-carpal joint may develop
- **C** there may be an associated avascular necrosis of the distal fragment
- **D** fusion of the wrist joint may be indicated when degenerative osteoarthritis develops
- **E** bone grafting is indicated when pain and instability are present without evidence of degenerative osteoarthritis

273 Concerning non-union of an uncomplicated tibial fracture treated in a plaster

- **A** Cortical bone graft is strong with good osteogenic potential
- **B** Cancellous bone graft is weak with good osteogenic potential
- **C** Hypertrophic fragment ends with plenty of callus formation suggest excessive movement at the fracture site which could be treated by internal fixation
- **D** An autogenous cortical bone graft is incorporated at the fracture site and remains viable
- **E** A bone inducing hormone has been identified which may be used instead of a bone graft to induce fracture healing

274 Dislocation of the sternoclavicular joint

- **A** is more common than dislocation of the acromio-clavicular joint
- **B** most commonly results in upwards and forward displacement of the medial end of the clavicle
- **C** is frequently unstable after reduction
- **D** may damage the trachea and great vessels if the dislocation is posterior
- **E** with marked displacement, indicates rupture of the costo-clavicular ligaments

Answers

272 A **True**
B **True**
C **False**
D **True**
E **True**

Non-union of a scaphoid fracture is a recognised complication. It may result after treatment of an acute injury or may be first seen as a long standing problem in a patient who has never presented with an acute injury. If the non-union is an incidental finding without symptoms, it is probably best left alone. If it follows an acute injury without evidence of osteo-arthritis but is causing pain and wrist instability, a bone graft is the treatment of choice. A non-union associated with radio-carpal arthritis may be treated by a silastic scaphoid replacement, or in a heavy manual worker, by fusion of the wrist.

273 A **False**
B **True**
C **True**
D **False**
E **False**

In fractures where there appears to be abundant callus formation at the fracture site excessive movement is usually the cause of non-union. Internal fixation by an intramedullary nail or plate and screws will produce rigidity and allow the callus to bridge and unite the fracture. In fractures with very little callus formation and resorption of bone, some method of stimulating osteogenesis is necessary. This usually takes the form of an autogenous bone graft. Cancellous bone which is very vascular and cellular is ideal but has no intrinsic strength. Cortical bone is strong, but does not have the potential for osteogenesis since it is relatively avascular and relatively acellular. The graft appears to induce the host bone cells to form bone but the trabeculae and osteocytes within the graft die and are resorbed. While there may be a bone inducing hormone present within the grafts, this has never been proven.

274 A **False**
B **True**
C **True**
D **True**
E **True**

Dislocation of the sterno-clavicular joint is less common than acromio-clavicular dislocations. It is caused by an indirect injury such as a fall on the outstretched hand, or in the case of posterior dislocations, direct injury. The more common anterior dislocation with rupture of the costo-clavicular ligaments results in the medial end of the clavicle lying anterior and upward due to the pull of sternomastoid. In the rare case of posterior dislocation, the great vessels and trachea may be compressed and urgent reduction is necessary. Either dislocation may be unstable after reduction and may require stabilisation using wire fixation.

Questions (*Answers overleaf*)

275 Concerning tarso-metatarsal dislocation

- **A** Lateral shift of the metatarsals will occur in an eversion injury
- **B** Complications include permanent stiffness and pain in the foot
- **C** Prompt reduction is advised to avoid the risk of permanent circulatory impairment
- **D** Open reduction is invariably necessary in dislocations without a fracture of the metatarsals
- **E** Avascular necrosis of the cuboid is a recognised complication

276 Injury to the brachial plexus may be caused by

- **A** an anterior dislocation of the shoulder
- **B** distraction of the head and shoulder
- **C** infiltration by a malignant tumour
- **D** a penetrating knife wound into the supraclavicular fossa
- **E** spontaneous pneumothorax

277 Fat embolus syndrome is associated with the following signs and symptoms

- **A** A pyrexia
- **B** Multiple lower limb fractures
- **C** Petechial haemorrhages
- **D** Pericarditis
- **E** A bradycardia

Answers

275 A **True**
B **True**
C **True**
D **False**
E **False**

Tarso-metatarsal dislocations are uncommon. There is frequently a history of a twisting injury to the foot in which the forefoot is everted or inverted on the hindfoot. Prompt reduction is advised since the circulation distal to the dislocation, especially the dorsalis pedis and medial plantar anastomosis, may be arrested. In a pure dislocation, closed reduction is usually simple, but in a fracture-dislocation, open reduction may be necessary and the position held with Kirschner wires. Despite adequate treatment, some patients develop stiffness and pain at the tarso-metatarsal joints due to degenerative arthritis.

276 A **True**
B **True**
C **True**
D **True**
E **False**

Brachial plexus injuries are frequently caused by a fall from a motor bike. The patient hits his shoulder and head against the ground and his head is then distracted laterally resulting in a traction injury to the plexus. More uncommon causes include an anterior dislocation of the shoulder resulting again in traction on the plexus. An infiltrating malignant tumour occasionally produces a plexus lesion. Two iatrogenic causes include accidental injury during excision of supraclavicular lymph glands and occasionally injury to the plexus during repair of a recurrent dislocation of the shoulder. Prolonged traction on the plexus during general anaesthesia, caused by poor positioning of the patient, is another preventable cause.

277 A **True**
B **True**
C **True**
D **False**
E **False**

The signs and symptoms of fat embolus syndrome include a tachycardia, tachypnoea and hypotension. There may be a sudden alteration in the patient's mental state including apprehension, restlessness or coma. On examination petechial haemorrhages may be seen in the conjuctivae, chest wall and anterior axillary folds. The syndrome usually occurs a few hours or several days after severe injury which often includes multiple lower limb fractures.

Questions (*Answers overleaf*)

278 On investigation, a patient with fat embolus syndrome is likely to have the following

A A 'snow storm' appearance on the chest radiograph
B An above normal arterial oxygen tension
C Fat globules in the urine
D A low arterial carbon dioxide tension
E Left heart strain on electrocardiogram

279 A complete traction injury of the lateral cord of the brachial plexus will result in

A paralysis of biceps and brachialis
B paralysis of the triceps muscle
C paralysis of the wrist dorsiflexors
D absent sensation over the palmar aspect of the little finger
E paralysis of the intrinsic muscles of the hand

280 Which of the following are indications for hemiarthroplasty in the shoulder and hip joint?

A A comminuted fracture of the head of the humerus in a 70 year old female
B A displaced subcapital fracture of the femur in a 30 year old male
C A fracture-dislocation of the head of the humerus in a 40 year old female
D A displaced subcapital fracture in a 70 year old female
E A displaced intertrochanteric fracture in a 75 year old female

281 Concerning the structures in the palmar surface of the wrist

A The radial artery lies to the radial side of the flexor pollicis longus
B The median nerve lies to the ulnar side of the flexor carpi radialis
C Flexor digitorum profundus lies superficial to the flexor digitorum sublimis
D The ulnar nerve and artery lie to the radial side of flexor carpi ulnaris
E Palmaris longus, although a vestigial tendon and muscle, is present in nearly all patients

Answers

278 A **True** B **False** C **True** D **False** E **False**

The positive investigations in fat embolus syndrome include a chest radiograph which may show the classical snow storm appearance and an ECG which may show right heart strain. Blood gas analysis will show a low arterial oxygen tension, often less than 60 mmHg. The patient may have a normal arterial carbon dioxide tension or hypercapnia. Urine analysis may show the presence of fat globules which may also be seen in the retinal vessels.

279 A **True** B **False** C **False** D **False** E **False**

An injury to the lateral cord will include paralysis of the biceps and brachialis (musculo-cutaneous nerve). Triceps and the wrist dorsiflexors are supplied by the posterior cord (radial nerve), the intrinsic muscles of the hand by the medial cord (ulnar and median nerves). Sensation to the plamar aspect of the little finger is through the medial cord (ulnar nerve).

280 A **True** B **False** C **False** D **True** E **False**

The two main factors when considering a hemiarthroplasty for intra-articular trauma are the complications of the prosthesis compared to the likelihood of complications if the constituents of the joint are preserved. A hemiarthroplasty has inherent complications including loosening, delayed infection, breakage and protrusio acetabuli in the case of the hip joint. In the younger the patient, there is a higher risk that one of these complications will develop and therefore it is better to maintain the original joint fragments and await events. In older patients with a limited life span, a definitive arthroplasty will result in improved function without a great risk of long term complications.

281 A **True** B **True** C **False** D **True** E **False**

Knowledge of the anatomy of the palmar aspect of the wrist is important in lacerating injuries. From radial to ulnar sides of the wrist lie the radial artery, flexor carpi radialis with flexor pollicis longus deep to it, palmaris longus with the median nerve deep to it, flexor digitorum superficialis with profundus deep to it, the ulnar artery and ulnar nerve, flexor carpi ulnaris. Palmaris longus tendon is absent in about 30% of patients.

Questions (*Answers overleaf*)

282 Tetanus
- **A** is caused by a Gram-positive organism, *Clostridium tetani*
- **B** produces a powerful neurotoxin
- **C** includes as a clinical feature paroxysmal muscle spasms
- **D** can be effectively treated by an intramuscular injection of anti-tetanus toxoid in an infected patient not previously immunised against tetanus
- **E** treatment in a non-immunised infected patient should include massive doses of penicillin and hyperimmune human gamma globulin

283 Complications of closed treatment of ankle fractures include
- **A** claw toes
- **B** non-union of the medial malleolus due to soft tissue interposition
- **C** persistent foot and ankle oedema
- **D** osteoarthritis of the ankle joint
- **E** subtalar stiffness

284 Two hours after treatment of a closed midshaft fracture of the tibia, the patient complains of persistent pain and numbness in the toes
- **A** The limb should be lowered below the level of the heart
- **B** The patient should be given increasing analgesia until pain is relieved
- **C** The plaster should be split down to skin along its whole length
- **D** The limb should be elevated
- **E** A chest radiograph should be ordered

Answers

282 A **True**
B **True**
C **True**
D **False**
E **True**

Tetanus is caused by infection with the spores of *Clostridium tetani* which form Gram-positive rods. The latter produce a powerful neurotoxin, tetanospasmin, which acts on the spinal cord to produce prolonged muscle contractions which are painful and caused by even mild stimuli. An infected patient not previously actively immunised against tetanus by antitetanus toxoid would not benefit from a toxoid injection since antibody takes time to develop. A non-immunised patient should receive massive doses of parenteral penicillin and passive immunity by injections of hyperimmune human gamma globulin.

283 A **True**
B **True**
C **True**
D **True**
E **True**

The closed treatment of ankle fractures is an accepted form of management providing accurate reduction is maintained until bony union. Complications include persistent foot and ankle oedema due to soft tissue injury and disuse. It may also be a manifestation of a deep venous thrombosis. Claw toes may occasionally occur due to fibrosis following ischaemia to muscles from a compartment syndrome. Non-union of a medial malleolar fracture is a recognised complication due to soft tissue interposition. Osteoarthritis of the ankle joint due to mal-union and articular cartilage damage at the time of injury may occur.

284 A **False**
B **False**
C **True**
D **True**
E **False**

The management of tibial fractures by plaster requires careful supervision to prevent complications which may markedly affect prognosis. Careful observation in the post-operative period is necessary and persistent pain at rest must be regarded with great suspicion. With rest and elevation, pain should not be a serious problem and its persistence suggests vascular compromise which should be relieved by completely splitting the plaster down to the skin. If not, then a compartment syndrome should be suspected in which the circulation to muscle is at risk from swelling within the confines of the fascial envelopes. Early decompression of the fascial compartments by operation will relieve symptoms and prevent muscle necrosis.

Questions (*Answers overleaf*)

285 A collar and cuff bandage would be suitable treatment for
- **A** an undisplaced fracture of the neck of the humerus
- **B** a displaced midshaft fracture of the humerus
- **C** a reduced dislocation of the elbow
- **D** a reduced Monteggia fracture in an adult
- **E** a crack fracture of the radial head

286 Gas gangrene following a soft tissue limb injury
- **A** is caused only by *Clostridium welchii*
- **B** is less likely to occur if an open skin wound with underlying muscle injury is sutured
- **C** is usually odourless
- **D** produces subcutaneous crackling as a classical physical sign
- **E** is invariably treated with large doses of intramuscular penicillin without the need for surgical debridement

287 A rugby player sustains a dislocation of the proximal interphalangeal joint of the ring finger
- **A** The dislocation is more frequently dorsal than palmar and is a hyperextension injury
- **B** Radiographs are of little value in management
- **C** After reduction of the dislocation, examination of the joint for stability is mandatory
- **D** Most dislocations are unstable after reduction and require some form of internal fixation
- **E** Following a stable reduction, garter strapping to the ring finger is all that is required

Answers

285 A **True**
B **False**
C **True**
D **False**
E **True**

A collar and cuff bandage supports the wrist against gravity, but allows longitudinal traction from the shoulder to the elbow. It cannot resist angular deformity of a long bone by itself and would be inappropriate treatment for a midshaft fracture of the humerus. It will maintain reduction of a fractured neck of humerus and an elbow dislocation providing the elbow is flexed above 90°. Similarly a crack fracture of the radial head could be treated by a collar and cuff since it rests the elbow, and allows contact between the articulating surfaces of the capitellum and the head. A Monteggia fracture, which is potentially unstable, could not be managed simply by a collar and cuff.

286 A **False**
B **False**
C **False**
D **True**
E **False**

Gas gangrene is caused by infection of a wound by *Clostridium welchii, septicum* and *oedematiens* which produce an odourless gas which passes along tissue planes to produce a crackling sensation as the examining hand presses on the infected tissue. These organisms prefer an anaerobic environment so that closed wounds are more at risk than those debrided and left open. The smell of gas gangrene due to tissue necrosis is revolting. Treatment is by wide excision of infected tissue up to the point where amputation may be necessary, together with massive doses of parenteral penicillin.

287 A **True**
B **False**
C **True**
D **False**
E **True**

Dislocations of the proximal interphalangeal joints of the fingers are usually hyperextension injuries resulting in dorsal displacement of the more distal phalanx. Radiographs are an important feature of management before reduction to exclude an intra-articular fracture and after manipulation to check reduction. Following reduction, examination of the joint for stability is essential, since an unstable joint requires a different post-reduction management to a stable joint. In a stable joint, early gentle mobilisation is acceptable whereas an unstable joint will require immobilisation or, depending on the presence of an intra-articular fracture, internal fixation.

Questions (*Answers overleaf*)

288 Concerning supracondylar fractures of the elbow in children

- **A** The distal fragment is displaced anteriorly more frequently than posteriorly
- **B** Cubitus varus deformity is invariably associated with joint stiffness
- **C** Cubitus valgus is more common than cubitus varus deformity
- **D** Neurological complications are usually transient
- **E** Permanent weakness of elbow flexion is a common sequel to the injury

289 A 20 year old patient is seen 6 weeks following an undisplaced Colles fracture. She complains of an inability to extend the metacarpophalangeal joint of the thumb and weakness of extension of the interphalangeal joint

- **A** The patient requires a psychiatric opinion
- **B** She has avulsed the extensor tendon of the thumb from the base of the distal phalanx
- **C** She has a partial injury to the posterior interosseous nerve which will recover spontaneously
- **D** Arrangements should be made to perform a tendon transfer to restore function of the long extensor of the thumb
- **E** The disability was probably present at the time of the original injury and should have been observed by the casualty officer

Answers

288 A **False** The majority of supracondylar fractures are caused
B **False** by a fall on the outstretched hand and result in
C **False** the distal fragment of the humerus being
D **True** angulated and displaced posteriorly. Much less
E **False** frequently, a direct injury to the elbow may result in forward angulation of the distal fragment. Following treatment, cubitus varus deformity is not uncommon and is due to persistant medial tilt of the distal fragment. Cubitus valgus deformity is a much rarer problem and usually of little cosmetic significance. The great majority of supracondylar fractures in children result in good or excellent function in the elbow and the deformity of cubitus varus is essentially a cosmetic problem. Most neurological problems are transient and are treated conservatively. Only if they fail to recover in the expected time should the nerve be explored.

289 A **False** Failure of a patient to extend the metacarpo-
B **False** phalangeal joint and weakness of extension of the
C **False** interphalangeal joint of the thumb is indicative of
D **True** a rupture of extensor pollicis longus which
E **False** classically occurs about 6 weeks following an undisplaced Colles fracture. Presumably it is an attrition rupture due to damage to the tendon at the extensor retinaculum and to ischaemia. Sometimes the patient notices very little disability, but in a young person transfer of extensor indicis to the long thumb extensor should be considered. Very occasionally, the rupture may heal spontaneously.

Questions (*Answers overleaf*)

290 Concerning a deep venous thrombosis in the lower limb

- **A** A diagnosis can always be made by clinical examination
- **B** A venogram is the most accurate method of diagnosis
- **C** Swelling of the calf following a total hip replacement is diagnostic of a deep venous thrombosis
- **D** Homan's sign is invariably positive in a thrombosis affecting the thigh
- **E** Tenderness over the affected segment of vein is a useful clinical sign

291 In traumatic central dislocations of the hip joint in a young adult

- **A** highly comminuted fractures of the acetabular floor without marked displacement of the femoral head should be treated conservatively
- **B** an isolated displaced fracture through the weight bearing portion of the acetabulum should be treated by open reduction and fixation
- **C** there may be an associated ipselateral midshaft femoral fracture
- **D** osteoarthritis is a common complication due to damage to the articular cartilage
- **E** permanent restriction of hip movement is uncommon following open reduction and internal fixation

Answers

290	A	**False**	Deep venous thrombosis is a common orthopaedic problem especially following surgery on the lower limbs. A high index of suspicion is necessary for diagnosis, since appropriate treatment may prevent a fatal pulmonary embolus. Unfortunately a diagnosis cannot always be made by clinical examination and the initial indication may be cardio-pulmonary collapse from an embolus. For this reason, some units use prophylactic anticoagulants post-operatively in high risk patients such as those undergoing total hip replacement. Clinical signs of a deep venous thrombosis include tenderness along the vein, swelling of the foot or calf and a positive Homan's sign when there is calf pain on dorsiflexion of the foot. In suspected patients, especially post-operatively, bilateral lower limb venograms will demonstrate the clot and allow appropriate treatment.
	B	**True**	
	C	**False**	
	D	**False**	
	E	**True**	
291	A	**True**	Central dislocations of the hip joint are usually caused by a force through the head of the femur being transmitted through the acetabulum. The aim of treatment is to reduce the fracture to its anatomical position and allow early hip movements. While it may be possible to treat these fractures surgically in isolated fractures through the floor of the acetabulum, surgery is not indicated in comminuted fractures and minimally displaced fractures and the fracture should be treated on Hamilton-Russell traction. Often, despite accurate reduction, articular damage is severe and degenerative osteoarthritis ensues. In fractures which have undergone open reduction and internal fixation, hip movements may be restricted. The force of the injury to the hip joint may also fracture the femoral shaft.
	B	**True**	
	C	**True**	
	D	**True**	
	E	**False**	

Questions (*Answers overleaf*)

292 Following transection of a peripheral nerve by a knife injury

A the axons and myelin sheaths fragment and degenerate proximally as far as the spinal cord
B the axons and myelin sheaths fragment distally along their whole length
C the axonal cell body takes no part in the response to injury
D the prognosis is better for mixed nerves rather than for a purely sensory or motor nerve
E providing the regenerated axon in the proximal stump enters the distal tube, it will pass along the tube at a rate of about 1 mm per day

293 Concerning simple and rapid clinical tests for the median and ulnar nerve function in the hand

A The abductor digiti minimi is supplied by the median nerve
B The skin on the palmar surface of the middle finger is invariably innervated by the median nerve
C The abductor pollicis brevis is supplied by the median nerve
D The skin of the little finger is supplied by the ulnar nerve
E The adductor pollicis muscle can be used as a simple test for the median nerve

Answers

292 A **False** B **True** C **False** D **False** E **True**

When a peripheral nerve is cut, the axons and myelin sheaths degenerate and fragment proximally for only a few millimetres. Distally, the whole length of the axon and myelin sheath degenerates (Wallerian degeneration). Macrophages and the Schwann cells clear the neural tube of debris. The cell body, either in the anterior horn for motor fibres, or the posterior root for sensory fibres, swell and the nissl granules consisting of endoplasmic retinculum and ribosomes undergo chromatolysis and disappear. The phase of axonal regeneration then occurs in which Schwann cells in the distal neural tube proliferate and if they are able to cross the gap, join the proximal tube. Regenerated axon sprouts then pass across to the distal tube and grow at a rate of about 1 mm per day. Prognosis is better in purely motor or sensory nerves and when the cut ends of the nerve are closely apposed without tension.

293 A **False** B **False** C **True** D **True** E **False**

There are many clinical situations when a rapid clinical check on median and ulnar nerve function in the hand is necessary, without resorting to time consuming fine tests. For sensory testing, light touch will provide information on the gross state of hand innervation. The skin of the little finger is invariably supplied by the ulnar nerve, while the palmar skin of the index finger is supplied by the median nerve. For testing the muscle function of the median and ulnar nerves, integrity of the abductor pollicis brevis muscle indicates an intact median nerve, whereas an intact abductor digiti minimi indicates an intact ulnar nerve. For comparison of one hand against the other, the muscles can be opposed and their relative strengths compared.

Questions (*Answers overleaf*)

294 Concerning fractures of the atlas and axis
- **A** Distraction and extension of the upper cervical spine can result in a fracture through the pedicles of the axis
- **B** A compression injury, such as a weight falling onto the skull, may result in a burst fracture of the ring of the atlas
- **C** Both of the above injuries invariably result in instantaneous death
- **D** A plain antero-posterior radiograph of the cervical spine is the most useful in identifying the fracture of the atlas
- **E** Tomograms of the upper cervical spine may be useful to identify the fractures

295 Concerning the anatomy of the front of the elbow
- **A** The brachial artery lies to the lateral side of the tendon of biceps brachii
- **B** The ulnar nerve passes posteriorly through the medial intermuscular septum and is not seen at the front of the elbow
- **C** The musculo-cutaneous nerve passes between brachialis and biceps brachii to form the posterior interosseous nerve
- **D** The median nerve passes beneath the two heads of pronator teres into the distal part of the forearm
- **E** The biceps tendon inserts into the medial side of the radius distal to the neck and is a powerful supinator of the forearm

296 Which of the following are correct?
- **A** A Galeazzi fracture is a fracture of the midshaft of the radius with an intact ulna and inferior radio-ulnar subluxation
- **B** A Hangman's fracture is a comminuted fracture of the ring of the atlas
- **C** A Maisonneuve fracture is a bimalleolar fracture of the ankle joint with displacement
- **D** A Dupuytren's fracture of the ankle is a fracture of the medial malleolus or rupture of the medial ligament, a fracture at the lower third of the fibula with tibio-fibular diastasis
- **E** Aviators astragalus is a stress fracture of the heel from prolonged flying

Answers

294 A **True** B **True** C **False** D **False** E **True**

A fracture through the pedicles of the axis, with or without displacement is either caused by distraction and extension of the neck or by compression and extension, when the drivers head hits the roof of a car in a road traffic accident. A compression injury may cause a burst fracture of the ring of the atlas with a variable amount of displacement. Surprisingly, not all patients with these types of fracture die, and they may present with either no neurological impairment or severe deficit. Whereas the pedicle fracture can usually be seen on the lateral radiograph of the cervical spine, the burst fracture is better visualised on the trans-oral film. In some cases, where radiographs are equivocal, tomograms of the region may be invaluable. More recently, CAT Scans have been used to provide further information on the severity of displacement of these fractures.

295 A **False** B **True** C **False** D **True** E **True**

The cubital fossa lies between pronator teres and brachioradialis and a line drawn between the humeral epicondyles contains the brachialis muscle in its floor. From the lateral to medial side it contains the radial and posterior interosseous nerves, the tendon of biceps which is inserted into the posterior part of the bicipital tuberosity of the radius, the brachial artery and the median nerve which passes out through the two heads of pronator teres. The musculo-cutaneous nerve, after giving off its muscular branches in the upper arm becomes the lateral cutaneous nerve of the forearm and pierces the deep fascia at the elbow.

296 A **True** B **False** C **False** D **True** E **False**

A Hangmans's fracture is a fracture of the axis through the pedicles with or without spondylolisthesis of the axis on C3. A Maisonneuve fracture is a fracture of the medial malleolus or rupture of the medial ligament, gross disruption of the interosseous membrane, diastasis of the tibia and fibula and a fracture of the fibula in the proximal third. A Dupuytren's fracture is the same injury, but the fibular fracture is in the lower third. Aviators astragalus is caused by sudden dorsiflexion of the foot when an aircraft crashes, resulting in a fracture through the neck of the talus.

Questions (*Answers overleaf*)

297 In a patient with a complete sciatic nerve palsy from a knife wound in the buttock

- **A** dorsiflexion of the foot will be normal
- **B** plantarflexion will be absent
- **C** extension of the knee will be weak
- **D** sensation over the plantar surface of the foot will be normal
- **E** the ankle jerk will be present

298 A patient sustains a spinal cord lesion in the midthoracic level resulting in transection of half of the spinal cord (Brown-Sequard lesion). The following neurological signs will be present distal to the lesion

- **A** Pain and temperature sense will be lost on the same side as the lesion
- **B** Position sense will be lost on the same side as the lesion
- **C** Vibration and deep pain sensation will be lost on the opposite side to the lesion
- **D** Motor function will be lost on the same side
- **E** There will be overflow incontinence of urine

299 A 'pulled' elbow

- **A** is a subluxation of the elbow joint
- **B** is a subluxation of the head of the radius from the annular ligament
- **C** results in classical changes on radiographs
- **D** usually requires manipulation under anaesthetic to relieve symptoms
- **E** most frequently occurs in children under 5 years of age

Answers

297 A **False** B **True** C **False** D **False** E **False**

The sciatic nerve supplies the hamstrings and all the muscles in the lower limb apart from the quadriceps, supplied by the femoral nerve and most of the adductors, supplied by the obturator nerve. The sciatic nerve divides into the tibial and peroneal nerves in the popliteal fossa. The former supplies the plantarflexors of the ankle before it passes into the foot as the medial and lateral plantar nerves. The common peroneal nerve supplies the peronei and the muscles in the extensor compartment of the leg and the muscle of extensor digitorum brevis in the foot. It also supplies the dorsal skin between the first and second toes. All the skin of the foot is supplied by branches of the sciatic nerve apart from the medial side of the foot and great toe which is supplied by the saphenous nerve; a branch of the femoral nerve.

298 A **False** B **True** C **False** D **True** E **False**

Following hemitransection of the spinal cord, the neurological signs distal to the lesion will depend on whether the fibres passing along the cord decussate and cross to the opposite half of the cord distal to the lesion. In the case of the posterior columns carrying fibres sensing position sense, deep pain and light touch and vibration sense they do not cross over and therefore will result in a deficit on the same side as the injury. The fibres in the lateral spino-thalamic tract carrying pain and temperature cross over to the opposite side of the cord near to their cell bodies, whereas the motor tracts pass downwards from the cerebrum on the same side of the cord having crossed over proximally in the medulla oblongata. Because the bladder has innervation from both sides of the spinal cord, it is not likely to be affected by the neurological deficit.

299 A **False** B **True** C **False** D **False** E **True**

A pulled elbow is a disorder mainly of the under 5 year olds in which the radial head slips under the annular ligament resulting in pain and restriction of rotation of the forearm. It usually occurs when the child's parent suddenly pulls the childs arm to prevent it running away. Often the symptoms subside spontaneously. In some patients gentle rapid rotation of the forearm into full supination and pronation will release the radial head. Radiographs are normal.

Questions (*Answers overleaf*)

300 External fixators for the treatment of fractures
- **A** are very useful in unstable fractures with serious soft tissue damage
- **B** are ideal for closed intra-articular fractures of the supracondylar region of the knee
- **C** may be complicated by pin-track infections
- **D** are never rigid enough to use without plaster support
- **E** do not allow compression of the fracture site

Answers

300 A **True** B **False** C **True** D **False** E **False**

External fixation devices in which pins are placed through the skin above and below a fracture and connected by clamps and metal rods have greatly enhanced treatment of fractures with soft tissue damage. The principle aim of the devices is to fix the fracture firmly, leaving the area of soft tissue damage free, to be treated as necessary. The device will hold a comminuted fracture out to length or will compress a stable fracture. The fixators are very strong and rigid when expertly applied. Complications include pin track infection and loosening of the pins. Closed intra-articular fractures are preferably treated by accurate reduction and internal fixation with screws and plates.